WORKBOOK

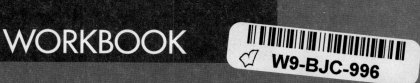

Health Science
Concepts and Applications

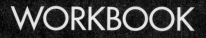

Publisher
The Goodheart-Willcox Company, Inc.
Tinley Park, IL
www.g-w.com

Cover Image: Caiaimage/Robert Daly/ Caiaimage/Getty Images

Contents

Chapter 1

Introduction to Healthcare Systems

Name _____ Date _____

Historical Contributions to Healthcare

Match each of the following advances in healthcare with the correct society, culture, or period in history from which they originated. Lettered items may be used more than once.

A. Ancient China	D. Romans	G. Renaissance
B. Ancient Egypt	E. Native Americans	H. Industrial Revolution
C. Ancient Greece	F. Dark and Middle Ages	I. Twentieth Century

_____ 1. Alexander Fleming discovered penicillin, the first antibiotic to treat bacterial infections.

_____ 2. Clara Barton formed the American Red Cross.

_____ 3. Maimonides described medical conditions, such as asthma and hepatitis, and emphasized the importance of a healthy lifestyle.

_____ 4. The invention of the stethoscope allowed doctors to listen more closely to a patient's heart and chest cavity.

_____ 5. The concepts of medicine and religion were separated.

_____ 6. The practice of acupuncture was developed.

_____ 7. DNA was discovered.

_____ 8. Scientists began using the scientific method.

_____ 9. Public health laws were established to help control the spread of disease.

_____ 10. Surgical instruments such as forceps and scalpels were invented.

_____ 11. Florence Nightingale demonstrated the critical role of nurses, hygiene, and nutrition in patient care.

_____ 12. Healers used herbs and natural pain relievers in the practice of medicine.

_____ 13. Marie and Pierre Curie discovered radium, which was later used in X-ray diagnostics.

_____ 14. The microscope was invented.

_____ 15. The concepts of diagnosis and prognosis were developed.

_____ 16. The pulse was first examined as an indicator of the severity of a disease.

_____ 17. Edward Jenner developed a smallpox vaccine.

_____ 18. The Hippocratic Oath was written.

_____ 19. Doctors first completed formal training and became licensed to practice medicine.

_____ 20. Cataract surgery was first performed.

Name _____ Date _____

Building Blocks from the Past

Throughout the years, many people have made major contributions to healthcare, and several of them are mentioned in chapter 1 of your textbook. Choose one of these people or someone else you know who has made a major contribution to healthcare. Research this person to find out more about his or her life, discoveries, and contributions to medical science. Write the information in the appropriate places on the graphic below. Then use this information to create a poster about the person.

Name of Contributor to Healthcare: _____

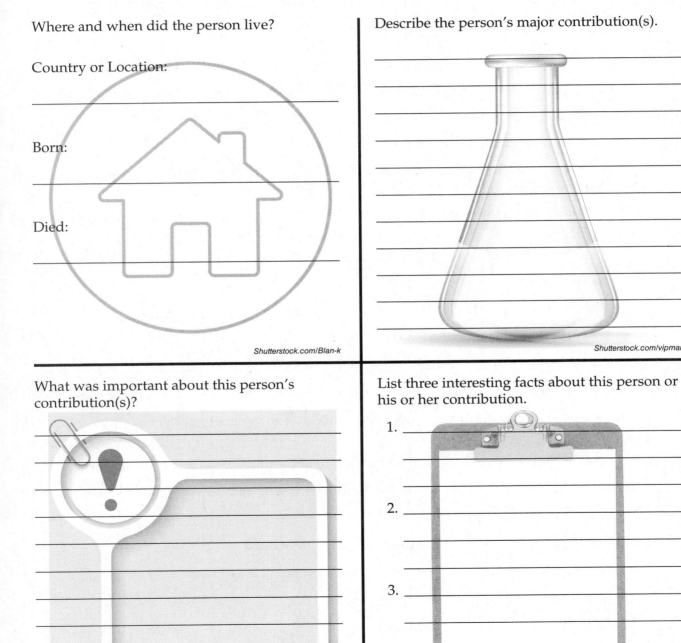

Where and when did the person live?

Country or Location:

_____

Born:

_____

Died:

_____

Shutterstock.com/Blan-k

Describe the person's major contribution(s).

Shutterstock.com/vipman

What was important about this person's contribution(s)?

Shutterstock.com/garriphoto

List three interesting facts about this person or his or her contribution.

1. _____

2. _____

3. _____

Shutterstock.com/Marie Maerz

Name _____ Date _____

Understanding Healthcare Terms

Use the terms listed here to fill in the blanks in the following statements. You will not use all of the terms.

anesthesia	deductible	hospice	premium	vaccination
antibiotics	epidemics	managed care	psychoanalysis	worker's
caduceus	genomic medicine	microscope	quarantine	compensation
copayment	Hippocratic Oath	pathogens	self-advocacy	

1. During the Dark Ages, millions of people were killed by _____ of the plague and other diseases for which there were no cures.

2. Government insurance that provides wage replacement and medical benefits for employees injured at work is known as _____.

3. HMOs and PPOs are examples of private organizations that are part of _____ insurance plans.

4. Early forms of _____, which causes a loss of feeling, included ether, nitrous oxide, and chloroform.

5. To maintain coverage under an insurance policy, the insured person pays a(n) _____ to the insurance company that issued the coverage.

6. The _____ is an emblem of medicine in the United States.

7. To build up a person's immunity to a specific disease, a(n) _____ containing weakened or dead bacteria or viruses may be administered.

8. A person under _____ has been isolated because he or she was exposed to an infectious or contagious disease.

9. Drugs called _____ are used to treat infections by slowing the growth of, or destroying, bacteria.

10. Terminally ill patients are often admitted to _____ facilities that focus on relieving their pain and symptoms.

11. Microorganisms that cause disease are known as _____.

12. In a(n) _____ session, a person who has a mental or emotional disorder is encouraged to talk about dreams and personal experiences.

13. The amount of money an insured person must pay annually for covered healthcare services before the health insurance plan begins to pay for those services is called the _____.

14. Protecting your own interests and making sure your needs are met are forms of _____, which requires you to make informed decisions about healthcare and other matters.

15. The branch of medicine that studies a person's DNA sequences to predict whether the person will contract a particular disease is called _____.

Medical Facilities Word Search

Search the grid of letters below for the terms listed in the word bank.

Word Bank

acute care	hospice	nonprofit	short-stay
dentist	hospital	optical	surgical center
dialysis	independent living	public	trauma center
doctor's office	long-term care	radiology	urgent-care center
for-profit	mental health	rehabilitation	walk-in clinic

```
W R Q T R H Y C L O L J E H F O I H D X Q P P T V
A E E T R V O E V A Q C K L Q N V V D W G K C F Z
L F C T Y A U S C W I U A K D G A J H V T F C S I
K X X S N F U R P F M M P E Z K L Q N Y N O Y Q N
I K K S K E L M F I E E P L O N G T E R M C A R E
N W A Y C A C O A N T E W L R R I I O K A X T E A
C A H Y Y X S L T C N A C K K I T C N N Q B S D O
L C T E E R G A A D E Y L I C T Y N D R H U T M B
I Z H I O C L Y E C H N S H G C K O B R U R R M X
N Y A T F H G N S I I S T K J D Q I C Z O P O W Y
I G C B E O T G S L I G D E L I F T X F T R H M T
C O O A K L R F D B B Z R J R A D A R P M H S H U
D A L S I E E P B U B S U U S L Z T V I X I F V N
G T G V P V Y Y V R P H U A O S Y I I G D G P R M Q
H G I R A D I O L O G Y Q D D S G L W L A U V X R
J N D I T H Z Z H D F E Q E X I T I J J E V S Q O
G P T I F O R P N O N Y N O H S E B V D R V U O O
E R E T N E C E R A C T N E G R U A E C X A S C K
J C G X Y B H R L N I L Z L A C I H O A O O G Z P
X G I G O Y J J U S T B P C Q W A E X G S S K I Z
O A F P L W H G T Z N Q E H V M R R O A B W U I O
K K C K S I H R H A L T U O S D J X N H P N J Z A
Z Q F J B O Q E Z A U N K B Z M K U V B N Y U W A
R D M J J D H M U C D D Y E B G Z C H W U F S P Q
L A C I T P O S A N R H G M F T B W Y A C L G G W
```

Making Sense of Insurance Options

People in the United States have many options for health insurance, and the best choice for one person or family is often not suitable for another. Read each description below and determine which type of public, government, or private insurance plan might be the best choice for the individual or family being described. Write the letter of the appropriate plan in the space provided. More than one answer may be valid for each description. Be ready to explain your choice in class.

MA: Medicaid

H: HMO

MC: Medicare

P: PPO

T: TRICARE

W: worker's compensation

_____ 1. A 30-year-old university student who served four years in the US Navy now works part-time while he earns a degree.

_____ 2. A single, 23-year-old woman is employed part-time, makes approximately $9,500 per year, and has two children ages 2 and 4.

_____ 3. In a nuclear family of five, with children ages 7, 9, and 13, the mother works in a home office, and the father has a job that requires frequent travel.

_____ 4. A 52-year-old engineer who has diabetes and takes insulin daily visits his healthcare provider several times a year for complications caused by diabetes.

_____ 5. A forklift driver was injured on the job when a stack of lumber fell on the forklift he was driving.

_____ 6. A 70-year-old retiree is currently living on Social Security and her company pension.

_____ 7. A 48-year-old man is self-employed and has a variable income that ranges from $10,000 to $60,000 per year, depending on how well his business thrives.

_____ 8. A 67-year-old woman is married to a retiree who fought in Vietnam.

_____ 9. A 32-year-old woman worked in a chemical laboratory until an accident in which a chemical compound caused an explosion that blinded her. She is no longer able to work.

_____ 10. A single, 56-year-old man works for a major manufacturing company, earning approximately $92,000 per year.

Debating the Affordable Care Act

The Affordable Care Act (ACA) has been controversial since it was passed in 2010. You may have heard people you know talk about how much they love or hate it. The two main issues the ACA has tried to address are access to healthcare for everyone and the affordability of healthcare. Choose one of these issues and conduct research to find out how the ACA addresses it. Be sure to use reliable, reputable sources in your research. For example, the US Department of Health and Human Services has a website dedicated to explaining the ACA. After studying your chosen issue, make an informed decision on whether the ACA has succeeded in addressing it. List your reasons below.

Compare notes with other students and form four debate teams based on your opinions. Two of the teams should debate whether the ACA has helped make healthcare more affordable. The other two teams should debate whether the ACA has helped make healthcare more accessible. While two teams are debating, the other two teams should form the audience for the debate and decide which team "wins."

Issue I researched: _____
_____

My informed opinion: _____
_____
_____
_____
_____
_____

My informed reasons: _____
_____
_____
_____
_____
_____
_____
_____
_____
_____
_____
_____

Chapter 2

Exploring Healthcare Careers

Name _____ Date _____

Matching Career Pathways

Match each of the following definitions with the correct career pathway term.

_____ 1. a two-year college degree awarded after completing 60 credit hours; commonly offered through a community college

_____ 2. the term for the progression from an entry-level position to a higher level of pay, skill, and responsibility

_____ 3. career pathway that offers many opportunities for hands-on experience and focuses on changing a patient's health status over time

_____ 4. highly scientific career pathway that uses living systems and organisms to create and develop products used in healthcare

_____ 5. a degree such as M.D., D.V.M., or Ph.D., which is awarded after two to six years of education beyond the bachelor's degree

_____ 6. recognition given for completing a scientific course of study and/or passing a specified exam

_____ 7. a healthcare career field considered to be a bridge between medicine and technology, which includes the management of health information and providing support to all other medical services

_____ 8. a system that categorizes patients according to their diagnoses

_____ 9. a healthcare pathway with careers involved in performing procedures to determine the causes of diseases or disorders

_____ 10. recognition given and required by a state agency; awarded when a person meets the qualifications for a particular occupation

_____ 11. a degree awarded after completion of one to two years of prescribed study beyond a bachelor's degree

_____ 12. a digital (computerized) record that contains information about a patient's medical history

_____ 13. occupations that play a critical role in healthcare, including the areas of safety, sanitation, equipment maintenance, counseling, marketing, and food preparation

_____ 14. a four-year college degree awarded after completing a minimum of 120 credit hours

_____ 15. a job exploration tool that involves following an employee while he or she completes the tasks of a job you find interesting

A. associate's degree

B. bachelor's degree

C. biotechnology research and development

D. career ladder

E. certificate

F. diagnostic-related groups (DRGs)

G. diagnostic services

H. doctorate degree

I. electronic health record (EHR)

J. health informatics services

K. job shadowing

L. licensure

M. master's degree

N. support services

O. therapeutic services

Understanding Healthcare Careers

Use the terms listed here to fill in the blanks in the following statements. You will not use all of the terms.

associate's degree	clinical internship	job shadowing	registered nurse
bachelor's degree	community college	licensure	support
biotechnology research and development	diagnostic	master's degree	technical
	electronic health records	Occupational Outlook Handbook	technician
career ladder			therapeutic
certification	health informatics	professional	

1. Following an employee while he or she completes the tasks of a particular job, known as _____, can be very helpful in finding a career you will find satisfying.

2. The clinical application of knowledge and skills previously learned in the classroom and laboratory is known as a(n) _____.

3. The _____ is a helpful online resource that can act as a starting point for career research.

4. Sometimes referred to as *vocational*, *trade*, or *proprietary* schools, _____ schools provide training for specific careers beyond high school.

5. A(n) _____ typically offers a two-year degree, called an *associate's degree*, in a specific course for a healthcare career.

6. After completing 60 credit hours or more in a college semester system, a(n) _____ is awarded.

7. Some healthcare careers require students to obtain a(n) _____, which is a four-year college degree awarded after completing 120 credit hours or more in a semester system.

8. An academic degree awarded for completing one to two years of prescribed study beyond the bachelor's degree is known as a(n) _____.

9. The healthcare employment level known as a(n) _____ often requires an associate's degree along with clinical training and possible licensure.

10. The _____ healthcare employment level requires a four-year or advanced degree as well as clinical training and possible licensure.

11. _____ is awarded by a state agency when a person meets the qualifications for a particular occupation and passes a required exam.

12. To recognize the completion of a specific course of study and/or passing a specified exam, _____ is given and can be voluntary or required according to the occupation.

13. The _____ services career pathway offers opportunities for hands-on experiences and focuses on changing the health status of a patient over time.

14. The progression from an entry-level position to higher levels of pay, skill, and responsibility is known as climbing the _____.

Healthcare Occupations Research

Follow the instructions in each step below to research health occupations that interest you.

1. Review the following list of healthcare occupations to determine the five careers that are most appealing to you at this time.

bioengineer	EMT/paramedic	optician
biological and chemical technician	health information specialist	optometrist
	health unit coordinator	pathologist
biomedical equipment technician	laboratory assistant	phlebotomist
	laboratory technician	physical therapist
clinical laboratory technologist	medical assistant	radiation oncologist
	microbiologist	radiation therapist
dentist	MRI technologist	radiologic technologist
diagnostic coding specialist	nuclear medicine technologist	radiologist
diagnostic medical sonographer		respiratory care worker
	occupational therapist	veterinarian
dietitian	ophthalmologist	

2. Now, research three of those careers using the Internet to discover the following information:

Job description: _____

_____

_____

Work environment: _____

_____

Education required: _____

_____

Licensure/certification required: _____

_____

Salary range: _____

Job outlook for the future: _____

_____

_____

(Continued)

Job description: _____

_____

_____

Work environment: _____

_____

Education required: _____

_____

Licensure/certification required: _____

_____

Salary range: _____

Job outlook for the future: _____

_____

_____

Job description: _____

_____

_____

Work environment: _____

_____

Education required: _____

_____

Licensure/certification required: _____

_____

Salary range: _____

Job outlook for the future: _____

_____

_____

3. Now, check the websites of local healthcare institutions for job opportunities in your area. Pay attention to job opportunities that align with the healthcare careers you researched. When you have found one job opportunity that interests you the most, create a short presentation about the job to share with the class. Be sure to include the information you listed here for this job.

Understanding Career Pathways

Match each of the following healthcare careers with the appropriate career pathway. You will use each career pathway more than once.

I.   therapeutic services career pathway
II. diagnostic services career pathway
III. health informatics services career pathway
IV. support services career pathway
V.   biotechnology research and development career pathway

_____ 1. microbiologist

_____ 2. radiation oncologist

_____ 3. pharmacist

_____ 4. central/sterile supply technician

_____ 5. medical illustrator

_____ 6. EKG technician

_____ 7. registered nurse

_____ 8. food services worker

_____ 9. medical records clerk

_____ 10. EMT

_____ 11. athletic trainer

_____ 12. biotechnological engineer

_____ 13. medical office manager

_____ 14. cytologist

_____ 15. biomedical equipment technician

_____ 16. radiologist

_____ 17. human resources technician

_____ 18. biological scientist

_____ 19. certified nursing assistant

_____ 20. registered dietitian

_____ 21. physician

_____ 22. research laboratory technician

_____ 23. diagnostic medical sonographer

_____ 24. director of support/central services

_____ 25. physician assistant

_____ 26. phlebotomist

_____ 27. registered health information technician

_____ 28. radiologic technologist

_____ 29. occupational therapist

_____ 30. medical librarian

_____ 31. optometrist

_____ 32. chemical technician

_____ 33. respiratory therapist

_____ 34. central services technician

_____ 35. optician

_____ 36. human resources manager

_____ 37. biological technician

_____ 38. mental health counselor

_____ 39. clinical laboratory technologist

_____ 40. dietetic technician

Name _____   Date _____

Healthcare Careers Word Search

Search the grid of letters below for the terms listed in the word bank.

associate's	doctorate	LVN	scientist
bachelor's	DRGs	master's	technician
biotechnology	health informatics	nursing	technologist
certification	EHR	optometrist	therapeutic
dentist	laboratory	pharmacist	X-ray
diagnostic	licensure	radiology	
doctor	LPN	RN	

```
A R T D E N G R I D B L M C O P D R B T U S D X R
G B E P C L R Y S A Z O E T V C I T S O N G A I D
N K C S H P N D O T I M R U B S W F Y V J E A R O
U B H Q G N I S R U N L M E X Y E H T E O B I Q U
E K N P R O T O Z I U R D T C S Y G O L O I D A R
M I I W X L P D R G S D C A U B N R L M E O H U C
L A C N H P U E X O E S I R T D E N T I S T C T T
O M I S U X S V Q D U T L O B R O K U S V E A E S
W U A S R O L E H C A B R T U N L E X S R C A C I
B O N V R I A L P Q V M S C Y R T N L T D H Q H R
L A B O R A T O R Y J A R O E N L T I L V N S N T
Q L G B E D T P H S A U F D R L S F N X I O R O E
Z P M T X I H M W K U D V K I I S E L T L C L M M
R H O M C E L E W I N A T N U C A C N L C O E O O
U A O V A L E N R S L T C N A T I L E I S G O G T
M R P T R S U T H R A N O T U T C E T N K Y R I P
C M O R S H T A E O B T I N S W B U L O S E T S O
K A V I G C L E Z T V O L I R E E H Y Q F U L T A
U C P L A R R B R L N E T I X P B O L T N E R Z K
T I R C O A N E T S N N P R A X O H Z R B M D E H
H S O T C E L I A V E S Q R A S S O C I A T E S L
X T T L E S C U J I U T E X R A D I L Y B Y M P A
C Y C W O E T E C O L H R E A H R W N Z O Y E S T
Y N O P S R N S C I T A M R O F N I H T L A E H S
R A D V Y M O A G E Y Q L Z M T E B I X A R N L T
```

Healthcare Career Pathways Bingo

Each of the five columns below is headed by the first letter of one of the five healthcare career pathways. List an appropriate career of your choosing in each square. For example, choose five therapeutic (T) careers and list one in each square beneath the letter "T." Do this for all five of the career pathways. Once you have filled every box, your teacher will call out occupations from the list below. If she calls out an occupation that appears in your bingo grid, place a mark in the appropriate box. The first student to get five connecting squares in a row is the winner.

athletic trainer
biological scientist
biological technician
biomedical equipment
   technician
biotechnological
   engineer
central/sterile supply
   technician
central services technician
certified nursing
   assistant
chemical technician

clinical laboratory
   technologist
cytologist
diagnostic medical
   sonographer
dietetic technician
director of support/
   central services
EKG technician
EMT
food services worker
human resources
   manager

human resources
   technician
medical illustrator
medical librarian
medical office manager
medical records clerk
mental health counselor
microbiologist
occupational therapist
optician
optometrist
pharmacist

phlebotomist
physician
physician assistant
radiation oncologist
radiologic technologist
radiologist
registered dietitian
registered health infor-
   mation technician
registered nurse
research laboratory
   technician
respiratory therapist

T	D	H	S	B
		FREE SPACE (OPTIONAL)		

Chapter 3

Healthcare Laws and Ethics

Name _____ Date _____

Law Versus Ethics

Read each of the following scenarios and determine whether the issue is a violation of the law, an ethical question, or both. Write the appropriate letter in the space provided. Then suggest a potential solution for the situation or a better course of action the healthcare worker should have taken.

L = Law

E = Ethics

B = Both

_____ 1. Cindy is a phlebotomist working the morning shift at the local hospital. Though she is normally well rested and ready for work, this morning she is feeling tired and irritable. Her 2-year-old son had a stomachache and kept her up most of the night. Her first patient is a 22-year-old male with a bad attitude. When she attempts to explain that she is going to obtain blood for testing, he sneers at her and asks, "You and what army?" Cindy snaps back at him, "I didn't order these tests, your doctor did. Now, hold still!"

Suggestions: _____

_____

_____

_____

_____

_____

_____

_____ 2. David is a newly hired medical assistant at New Hope Clinic. During his second day on the job, he notices one of the other medical assistants slip a pharmaceutical sample box of a prescription antacid into his lab coat pocket before leaving for the day. David is unsure of what to do.

Suggestions: _____

_____

_____

_____

_____

_____

_____

(Continued)

_____ 3. A doctor is treating Mario, a patient who is dying of lung cancer. Neither chemotherapy nor radiation has been successful in treating his cancer, and Mario is now a hospice patient with less than six months to live. Mario, who is obviously in great pain in spite of heavy doses of painkillers, begs the doctor to "help me end it." The doctor writes a prescription for a large quantity of oral morphine and tells the patient, "It's up to you how much of this you take at one time."

Suggestions: _____

_____

_____

_____

_____

_____

_____

_____ 4. Li, an ECG technician, has tried to explain to her elderly male patient that an ECG will not send harmful electricity through his body. The patient flatly refuses to believe her, and he will not allow her to perform the ECG. Li reports this to her supervisor, who asks Michel, another ECG technician on staff, to explain the procedure to the patient. When Michel approaches the patient, the patient says, "That other technician doesn't know what she is talking about!" In an attempt to calm the patient, Michel answers, "Yes, I agree. She has a reputation for that." The patient finally agrees to allow the ECG to be performed.

Suggestions: _____

_____

_____

_____

_____

_____

_____

Understanding Legal Principles in Healthcare

Use the terms listed here to fill in the blanks in the following statements.

advance directive	defamation	invasion of privacy	reasonable care
arbitration	durable power of attorney	libel	scope of practice
assault		malpractice	slander
battery	duty of care	negligence	standard of care
confidentiality	emancipated minor guardian	ombudsman	statute of limitations

1. A healthcare worker's legal obligation to take reasonable care of a patient to avoid causing harm is called _____.

2. The practice of resolving legal disputes without going to court, called _____, can help protect a healthcare facility from the expenses associated with going to trial.

3. After bathing a hospitalized patient, the nursing assistant did not raise the bed rails on the hospital bed. Half an hour later, the patient rolled over and fell out of the bed. This is an example of _____ on the part of the nursing assistant.

4. Protecting the legal rights of a patient and ensuring that the patient is not abused are duties of a(n) _____.

5. The concept of _____ involves the protection of a patient's personal and health-related information so that only professionals who need the information have access to it.

6. A(n) _____ can be either physical or informational.

7. The amount of time during which a person can bring a lawsuit against another person or company is known as the _____.

8. The act of damaging someone's good name or reputation either verbally or in writing is known as _____.

9. Mrs. Whitman has been legally declared incompetent because she has advanced dementia. The court may appoint a(n) _____ to make decisions for Mrs. Whitman and protect her interests.

(Continued)

10. An EMT has been ordered by the ER doctor to obtain a blood sample from a woman who was involved in a car accident. The woman refuses to cooperate, so the EMT grabs her arm and attempts to hold it steady so that he can obtain the blood sample. This is an example of

    _____.

11. A surgeon performing routine gallbladder surgery slips, and the scalpel nicks the patient's pancreas, causing internal bleeding for weeks after the surgery. This is an example of

    _____ on the part of the surgeon.

12. Karen, an RN at a teaching hospital, has been asked to help introduce a newly hired RN to the hospital's policies and procedures. After a long and trying day, she posts about the new RN on Facebook, saying that "Mr. K. has the mentality of an average two-year-old." Karen is guilty of

    _____.

13. Many hospitals and other healthcare facilities require patients to have a(n) _____, which is a legal document that gives specific instructions about healthcare decisions to be used if the patient becomes incapable of making those decisions.

14. Sonja is 17 years old, but she has been living on her own for more than a year. She is considered a(n) _____ and is legally and financially responsible for herself.

15. The principle of _____ specifies that healthcare practitioners must perform a procedure in the same way that someone with similar qualifications would have performed it under similar circumstances.

16. If it is proven that a healthcare worker acted reasonably as compared to other members of the profession in the same or a similar situation, the legal protection known as

    _____ can be used.

17. A(n) _____ grants another person the authority to make legal decisions for you.

18. During a patient exam, Dr. Fairbanks corrects his nurse, Alice, on part of her job. Alice feels embarrassed and is angry with Dr. Fairbanks. At lunch, Alice tells a coworker, "Dr. Fairbanks is totally unqualified for his position." Alice is guilty of _____.

19. If a healthcare worker argues with a patient who does not want a procedure, it may be considered _____.

20. A healthcare worker's _____ includes all the skills she is trained for and allowed to use.

Applying a Code of Ethics

Many professional organizations for healthcare workers have a code of ethics that all members are expected to follow. The code of ethics for the American Association of Medical Assistants (AAMA) is shown here. Read the code carefully, and then answer the questions that follow.

AAMA Code of Ethics

Members of AAMA dedicated to the conscientious pursuit of their profession, and thus desiring to merit the high regard of the entire medical profession and the respect of the general public which they serve, do pledge themselves to strive always to:

A.   Render service with full respect for the dignity of humanity.

B.   Respect confidential information obtained through employment unless legally authorized or required by responsible performance of duty to divulge such information.

C.   Uphold the honor and high principles of the profession and accept its disciplines.

D.   Seek to continually improve the knowledge and skills of medical assistants for the benefit of patients and professional colleagues.

E.   Participate in additional service activities aimed toward improving the health and well-being of the community.

American Association of Medical Assistants

---

1. Give at least two examples of how a healthcare professional could fulfill item A in the code of ethics. Be specific.

   _____

   _____

   _____

   _____

   _____

   _____

2. Explain what is meant by "respect confidential information" in item B. Give an example of how this can be achieved.

   _____

   _____

   _____

   _____

   _____

   _____

(Continued)

3. Item E of the code does not relate directly to patient care or even to the workplace. How does this item apply to a healthcare worker's ethics?

_____

_____

_____

_____

_____

_____

_____

_____

_____

_____

4. Use the Internet to find a code of ethics for another healthcare-related professional organization. Compare that code of ethics with the one shown here. Write a paragraph describing the similarities and differences between the two codes of ethics.

_____

_____

_____

_____

_____

_____

_____

_____

_____

_____

_____

_____

Interpreting the HIPAA Privacy Rule

The following excerpt is from a summary of the HIPAA Privacy Rule provided by the US Department of Health and Human Services. Read the excerpt carefully. Look up any words you do not know. Then write a summary of this information using language that the average middle school student would understand. In your summary, be sure to explain the difference between protected health information and de-identified health information.

Protected Health Information. The Privacy Rule protects all *"individually identifiable health information"* held or transmitted by a covered entity or its business associate, in any form or media, whether electronic, paper, or oral. The Privacy Rule calls this information "protected health information (PHI)."

"Individually identifiable health information" is information, including demographic data, that relates to:

- the individual's past, present or future physical or mental health or condition,
- the provision of health care to the individual, or
- the past, present, or future payment for the provision of health care to the individual,

and that identifies the individual or for which there is a reasonable basis to believe it can be used to identify the individual. Individually identifiable health information includes many common identifiers (e.g., name, address, birth date, Social Security Number).

The Privacy Rule excludes from protected health information employment records that a covered entity maintains in its capacity as an employer and education and certain other records subject to, or defined in, the Family Educational Rights and Privacy Act, 20 U.S.C. §1232g.

De-Identified Health Information. There are no restrictions on the use or disclosure of de-identified health information. De-identified health information neither identifies nor provides a reasonable basis to identify an individual. There are two ways to de-identify information; either: (1) a formal determination by a qualified statistician; or (2) the removal of specified identifiers of the individual and of the individual's relatives, household members, and employers is required, and is adequate only if the covered entity has no actual knowledge that the remaining information could be used to identify the individual.

_____

_____

_____

_____

_____

_____

_____

_____

_____

(Continued)

_____

_____

_____

_____

_____

_____

_____

_____

_____

_____

_____

_____

_____

_____

_____

_____

_____

_____

_____

_____

_____

_____

_____

_____

_____

_____

_____

_____

_____

_____

_____

_____

_____

_____

_____

_____

_____

_____

Identifying Forms of Mistreatment

Review the definition of each term in the table below. Then read the statements that follow. Place the number of each statement under the term that best identifies the type of mistreatment the patient is experiencing in that situation. Some statements may fit into more than one category.

Abuse	Assault	Battery	Invasion of Privacy	Malpractice	Negligence

1. A nursing assistant who is assigned to bathe a psychiatric patient uses unauthorized physical restraints to keep the patient still while she is working.

2. During a kidney transplant operation, the surgical team provides a woman who has O-positive blood with a kidney removed from a donor who has type A blood. The patient has a severe reaction and dies.

3. A physician assistant in the emergency room begins to place a blood pressure cuff on the arm of a car accident victim. Both of the patient's arms are bruised from the accident, and the patient requests that a blood pressure cuff not be used. The physician assistant insists that it is necessary and proceeds to use the blood pressure cuff against the patient's wishes, causing great pain.

4. A young mother brings her toddler into the reception area at the pediatrician's office. The toddler is in pain and is screaming loudly, upsetting the other patients. The parent of another patient approaches the mother, raises her hand, and says, "If you can't stop your child from crying, I can! All it takes is a good slap."

5. An appendectomy is performed on a 27-year-old patient, who later claims that the surgery was unnecessary. The medical staff had neglected to ask him to sign an informed consent form.

6. An 80-year-old woman is brought to the doctor's office by her daughter for a routine checkup. Every time the doctor asks the woman a question, her daughter answers for her. When the doctor asks the daughter to allow her mother to answer, the daughter says, "Oh, she's too old and stupid to understand."

7. A man is brought to the emergency room complaining of chest pain. The busy ER doctor determines that the cause is gastrointestinal reflux disease (GERD) and sends him home with instructions to change his diet. Three days later, the man has a massive heart attack and dies.

8. During her routine annual physical, a woman is newly diagnosed with high cholesterol. The doctor explains the different measures she can take to reduce her cholesterol level, and she decides to try modifying her diet instead of taking medication. Three weeks later, she begins receiving advertisements from various drug companies for cholesterol medications.

Name _____ Date _____

Scrambled Legal Terms

Unscramble the letters in each item below to form a legal term. Then define each term.

1. N A T A B O I T I R R

   Term: _____

   Definition: _____

2. L U V A S E

   Term: _____

   Definition: _____

3. M S U N A B M D O

   Term: _____

   Definition: _____

4. C H I E S T   T O T E M C I M E

   Term: _____

   Definition: _____

5. E T O F A D N I A M

   Term: _____

   Definition: _____

6. C E D A A N V   R E C E I V I D T

   Term: _____

   Definition: _____

7. M E T A P A I D E N C   O R I N M

   Term: _____

   Definition: _____

8. D A N A R I G U

   Term: _____

   Definition: _____

Chapter 4

Safety and Infection Control

Name _____   Date _____

Workplace Safety Terminology

Use the terms listed here to fill in the blanks in the following statements.

body mechanics

burn

carpal tunnel
  syndrome

disaster

ergonomics

fire triangle

hospital emergency
  codes

incident reports

MSDS (material safety
  data sheet)

OSHA Hazard
  Communication
  Standard

quality improvement
  (QI)

straight

1. _____ are signals used in hospitals to alert staff to fire, cardiac arrest, hazardous material, bomb threat, and other emergencies.

2. A(n) _____ is any sudden event that brings great damage, loss, or destruction, for which all individuals in the healthcare profession must be prepared at all times.

3. The forms used in a healthcare facility to document both safety- and non-safety-related events that are not part of a routine operation in the facility are known as _____.

4. The _____, established by the Occupational Safety and Health Administration, requires employers to educate employees about chemical hazards in the workplace.

5. The most common chemical injury is a(n) _____.

6. A(n) _____ contains comprehensive information about a particular chemical's makeup, dilution and mixture concentration, and instructions for use.

7. The three elements needed to start and maintain a fire—fuel, heat, and oxygen—are known as the

   _____.

8. The proper use of body movements to prevent injury during the performance of physical tasks such as lifting and sitting is known as _____.

9. _____ is the practice or science of maximizing efficiency and preventing discomfort or injury during the time a person is performing work-related tasks.

10. A progressively painful hand and arm condition known as _____ can be prevented by maintaining a proper wrist position while operating a computer keyboard.

11. When lifting a heavy object, you should lift with your legs and keep your back

    _____ at all times.

12. _____ policies motivate or require healthcare facilities to monitor and evaluate their services based on predetermined criteria for the purpose of improving those services.

Name _____ Date _____

Identifying Laboratory Safety Symbols

Identify each of the following laboratory safety symbols. Then provide a description of what each symbol represents, as well as the potential hazards associated with each one.

	Symbol: **Description:** **Associated Hazards:**
	Symbol: **Description:** **Associated Hazards:**
	Symbol: **Description:** **Associated Hazards:**
	Symbol: **Description:** **Associated Hazards:**
	Symbol: **Description:** **Associated Hazards:**
	Symbol: **Description:** **Associated Hazards:**
	Symbol: **Description:** **Associated Hazards:**
	Symbol: **Description:** **Associated Hazards:**
	Symbol: **Description:** **Associated Hazards:**
	Symbol: **Description:** **Associated Hazards:**

Ecelop/Shutterstock.com; Max Griboedov/Shutterstock.com; andromina/Shutterstock.com; Miguel Angel Salinas Salinas/Shutterstock.com; Barry Barnes/Shutterstock.com

Which Class of Fire Extinguisher?

Match each of the following materials with the correct class of fire extinguisher that would be used in a fire involving that material. Each class of fire extinguisher may be used more than once. Some materials may have more than one correct class of fire extinguisher.

A: class A
B: class B
C: class C
D: class D
E: classes A, B, and C

_____ 1. gasoline

_____ 2. magnesium

_____ 3. paper

_____ 4. wiring

_____ 5. wood

_____ 6. sodium

_____ 7. grease

_____ 8. computers

_____ 9. potassium

_____ 10. textiles (fabric)

_____ 11. paints

_____ 12. titanium

_____ 13. oils

_____ 14. energized electrical equipment

_____ 15. flammable liquids

_____ 16. combustible metals

_____ 17. ordinary combustibles

_____ 18. flammable materials requiring carbon dioxide to extinguish

_____ 19. flammable materials requiring a dry chemical extinguisher

_____ 20. materials requiring pressurized water (only) to extinguish

Name _____ Date _____

Using Proper Body Mechanics

One of the most important guidelines of personal safety in a workplace is the use of proper body mechanics. Healthcare workers are required to lift and move objects on a daily basis, so they must use proper ergonomic practices to limit personal injuries. In the space provided below, list the steps (in order) for properly lifting a 15–20 pound box from the floor, moving it to another location across the room, and setting it down.

_____

_____

_____

_____

_____

_____

_____

_____

_____

_____

_____

_____

_____

_____

_____

_____

_____

_____

_____

_____

_____

_____

_____

_____

Safety and Quality Improvement in the Healthcare Workplace

Answer the following questions.

1. List 10 general or standard safety rules that should be found in the safety manual of a healthcare facility.

   _____

   _____

   _____

   _____

   _____

   _____

   _____

   _____

   _____

   _____

   _____

2. Provide six examples of frequently used hospital emergency codes. Explain the threat that is represented by each code.

   _____

   _____

   _____

   _____

   _____

   _____

   _____

   _____

   _____

   _____

3. Why do hospitals use emergency codes instead of announcing specific emergencies?

   _____

   _____

   _____

   _____

   _____

   _____

   _____

(Continued)

4. Draw five laboratory safety symbols and explain what each one represents.

5. List and briefly describe the 10 universal guidelines for patient safety.

_____

_____

_____

_____

_____

_____

_____

_____

_____

_____

6. What precautions should you take when entering a patient's room and leaving a patient's room?

_____

_____

_____

_____

_____

_____

_____

_____

_____

_____

(Continued)

7. What should you do if a patient refuses treatment or refuses to allow you to perform your work duties?

_____

_____

_____

_____

8. What types of situations should be documented on an incident report?

_____

_____

_____

_____

9. What does the acronym *ALARA* mean? What three factors does ALARA take into account?

_____

_____

_____

_____

10. What does the fire triangle represent?

_____

_____

11. Briefly describe each of the three classifications or degrees of burns.

_____

_____

_____

_____

_____

12. Indicate the proper order in which bedridden patients, ambulatory patients, and wheelchair patients should be evacuated in the event of a fire emergency.

_____

_____

_____

_____

(Continued)

13. What does the acronym *PASS* mean in relation to the proper use of a fire extinguisher?

_____

_____

_____

14. List 10 principles of good body mechanics that should be used when lifting objects.

_____

_____

_____

_____

_____

_____

_____

_____

_____

_____

_____

_____

_____

_____

_____

_____

15. Briefly describe each of the following governmental agencies that are involved in protecting the health and safety of patients and the public.

FDA: _____

_____

NIH: _____

_____

CDC: _____

_____

TJC: _____

_____

WHO: _____

_____

Name _____   Date _____

Infection Control Terminology

Match each of the following definitions with the correct term.

A. aerobe	G. biohazard	K. direct contact	Q. MRSA
B. anaerobe	sharps container	L. disinfection	R. morphology
C. antisepsis	H. biopsy	M. fungi	S. needlesticks
D. asepsis	I. bloodborne	N. indirect contact	T. Needlestick
E. autoclave	pathogens	O. infection control	Safety and
F. bacteria	J. chain of infection	P. isolation rooms	Prevention Act

_____ 1. all of the activities involved in preventing the spread of infection

_____ 2. small, one-celled microorganisms that cannot be seen by the naked eye and which are potentially pathogenic

_____ 3. parasitic organisms, including disease-causing microorganisms such as yeasts and molds, that live in the soil or on plants

_____ 4. an organism that requires little or no oxygen to survive

_____ 5. an organism that requires an environment with oxygen to live

_____ 6. the science or study of the form and structure of organisms

_____ 7. an antibiotic-resistant bacterium responsible for an infection that is difficult to treat and is sometimes prevalent in hospitals, prisons, schools, and nursing homes

_____ 8. a type of infection transmission in which the pathogen takes an indirect path of transmission—such as through food, air, or clothing—to its next host

_____ 9. a type of infection transmission in which the pathogen travels directly from one host to another

_____ 10. the sequence of events that allows an infection to invade the human body, consisting of an infectious agent, reservoir or host, portal of exit, mode of transmission, portal of entry, and susceptible host

_____ 11. a term used to describe the absence of bacteria, viruses, and other microorganisms

_____ 12. the process of using an antiseptic to prevent or inhibit the growth of pathogenic organisms

_____ 13. the term used to describe the use of antimicrobial agents on nonliving objects or surfaces to destroy or deactivate microorganisms

_____ 14. an instrument or machine that uses hot, pressurized steam to kill all microorganisms and their spores on a surface

_____ 15. infectious microorganisms in human blood that can cause disease

_____ 16. the process of removing tissue for examination and diagnosis

_____ 17. rooms in a healthcare facility used to prevent the spread of infections, either by containing patients who have contagious diseases or by protecting immune-compromised patients from infectious diseases

_____ 18. any accidental punctures of the skin by needles, which can cause a potentially serious infection

_____ 19. a puncture-resistant container used for disposing of waste-contaminated sharps, including needles, scalpels, glass slides, and broken glassware

_____ 20. a law enacted in 2000 requiring employers to identify, evaluate, and introduce safer medical devices to avoid needlesticks

Understanding Infection Control

Use the terms listed here to fill in the blanks in the following statements.

bacteria

fungi

nosocomial infections

OSHA Bloodborne
    Pathogens Standard

parasites

personal protective
    equipment (PPE)

potentially infectious
    materials (PIM)

protozoa

rickettsiae

sanitization

sharps

standard precautions

sterilization

vectors

viruses

1. _____ are small, one-celled microorganisms that require a microscope to be seen.

2. Very small pathogenic organisms that depend on a living cell to survive are known as

   _____.

3. Parasitic organisms that live in the soil or on plants are called _____.

4. Microorganisms known as _____ may cause serious illnesses such as

   dysentery, trichomoniasis, and malaria.

5. _____ are parasites that normally choose fleas, lice, ticks, or mites as their

   host organisms and may cause severe infections such as Rocky Mountain spotted fever and typhus.

6. Infections acquired in hospitals and other healthcare facilities are known as

   _____, or *healthcare-acquired infections*.

7. Carriers known as _____ spread pathogens from one host to another and

   can include insects, rodents, and other small animals.

8. _____ is the use of antimicrobial agents on objects, surfaces, or living tissue

   to reduce the number of disease-causing microorganisms that are present.

9. Rickettsiae are an example of _____, which are known as organisms that

   live in or on another organism.

10. The act of destroying all microorganisms and their spores on a surface by using methods such as

    an autoclave is known as _____.

11. The Occupational Safety and Health Administration developed a set of guidelines known as the

    _____ to list potentially infectious materials and mandate that all health-

    care workers proceed at all times as if those materials are infectious.

12. _____ are substances such as blood, secretions, body fluids, and human

    tissue that require healthcare workers to proceed as if they are infectious.

13. A set of basic practices intended to prevent transmission of infectious diseases from one person to

    another are known as _____.

14. Equipment such as face shields, face masks, safety glasses, goggles, gowns, and gloves worn by

    workers to protect them from serious workplace injuries or illnesses are known collectively as

    _____.

15. Needles and any other _____ or objects that could puncture or cut the skin

    are a hazard in the healthcare environment.

The Chain of Infection

Nosocomial infections can be difficult to treat or overcome. The best way to deal with an infection is to prevent the infection from spreading from one person or area to another. The chain of infection is a helpful way to visualize the sequence of events that occur to allow an infection to be transmitted. In the space provided below, draw your own version of the chain of infection, including all of the components that make up the cycle, as described in your textbook.

Analyzing Hand Hygiene

Hand washing is considered to be the single most important way to prevent the spread of infection. Answer the following questions about hand washing, hand hygiene, and hand protection.

1. According to the CDC guidelines for healthcare workers, when should the hands be washed?

   _____

   _____

2. How long should the hands be washed to practice proper hand hygiene? What song is commonly sung during hand washing to ensure that the activity lasts long enough? Name another common song that you could use for this purpose.

   _____

   _____

3. Briefly list the steps involved in proper hand washing.

   _____

   _____

   _____

   _____

   _____

   _____

   _____

   _____

4. To protect your hands from exposure to potentially infectious materials, protective gloves should be worn. List the steps for properly putting gloves on your hands, and then list the steps for properly removing the gloves once they have been used.

   _____

   _____

   _____

   _____

   _____

   _____

   _____

   _____

5. Demonstrate proper hand washing and gloving techniques for your teacher if the proper equipment and supplies are available.

Medical and Surgical Asepsis

Identify each of the following aseptic techniques as being part of medical asepsis or surgical asepsis.

M = medical asepsis
S = surgical asepsis

_____ 1. using an autoclave

_____ 2. using an antiseptic

_____ 3. using a disinfectant

_____ 4. sanitizing the surface of a desk or table

_____ 5. using hot, pressurized steam to sterilize

_____ 6. using an alcohol-based substance to clean an object

_____ 7. using chemicals to kill all microorganisms without killing their spores

_____ 8. using dry heat, gas, or radiation to kill all microorganisms and their spores

_____ 9. using "clean technique"

_____ 10. using "sterile technique"

Answer the following questions.

11. What are the three levels of cleaning that take place in healthcare facilities to prevent the spread of pathogens? Briefly describe each one.

_____

_____

_____

_____

_____

_____

_____

_____

_____

_____

_____

_____

12. In a hospital, which department handles sterilization procedures?

_____

Analyzing Infection Control

Answer the following questions.

1. Provide one example of nonpathogenic microorganisms.

   _____

2. Name five different types of microorganisms that cause infectious diseases.

   _____

   _____

3. What is the difference between aerobes and anaerobes?

   _____

   _____

   _____

4. Name and draw 10 specific types of bacteria.

5. Which drugs kill disease-inducing microorganisms that cause bacterial infections?

   _____

6. Name five diseases caused by viruses.

   _____

   _____

7. How are viruses treated?

   _____

   _____

(Continued)

8. What is MRSA? Why is it called a *super bug*?

_____

_____

_____

9. What is the single most important method of preventing the spread of infection in a healthcare facility?

_____

10. Which term describes an infection acquired by a patient while he or she was in the hospital or another healthcare facility?

_____

11. Compare the terms *medical asepsis* and *surgical asepsis*.

_____

_____

_____

12. What is an autoclave?

_____

_____

13. According to recent research, which method of drying your hands is considered most hygienic?

_____

14. In which situations and on what types of patients would you use standard precautions?

_____

_____

15. Which practices are covered under the standard precautions?

_____

_____

_____

_____

16. Define *transmission-based precautions* and identify their three categories.

_____

_____

_____

(Continued)

17. List five types of personal protective equipment (PPE).

    _____

    _____

18. What types of items or equipment should be placed in a biohazard sharps container after being used on a patient?

    _____

    _____

19. Should needles be recapped before they are placed in a biohazard sharps container? Why or why not?

    _____

    _____

    _____

20. What procedure should be followed if you are stuck by a used needle or otherwise directly exposed to potentially infectious materials?

    _____

    _____

Chapter 5

Medical Terminology

Name _____ Date _____

Dissecting Medical Terms

Break each term in the following chart into its word elements. Write each element under the appropriate column. Some terms may include only some of the possible word elements. In the last column, define the term. Look up the term in a medical dictionary if you are not sure of its meaning.

Term	Prefix	Word Root/ Combining Form	Suffix	Definition
intravenous				
hypodermic				
transocular				
encephalitis				
myeloma				
neurology				
arthroscopy				
proctalgia				
ultrasound				
paresthesia				
gastric				
thrombolytic				

Name _____ Date _____

Medical Term Building Blocks

Use the word elements in the image shown here to create terms that match each definition below. Some word elements may be used more than once, but you will not use all of the word elements. You may refer to a medical dictionary to complete this activity.

1. pertaining to around the eye:

   _____

2. process of cutting of a bone:

   _____

3. pain in the muscle:

   _____

4. surgical removal of the appendix:

   _____

5. inflammation of the pancreas:

   _____

6. incision into the iris of the eye:

   _____

7. surgical repair of the eardrum:

   _____

8. visual examination of the abdomen using
   a scope: _____

9. pertaining to against itching:

   _____

10. pertaining to the breakdown or destruction
    of blood: _____

11. inflammation of the nail:

    _____

12. condition of losing color in the skin:

    _____

tympan/o	anti-	-ation	oste/o
peri-	ventricul/o	-scopy	-ary
arteri/o	ocul/o	-ic	hypo-
angi/o	irid/o	de-	append/o
pigment/o	onych/o	my/o	-stasis
-ectomy	-emia	-form	prurit/o
pancreat/o	hem/o	-itis	-sclerosis
lapar/o	atri/o	-plasty	axill/o
-algia	-prandial	-megaly	-ar
aur/i	-tomy	-lytic	

13. pertaining to the atria and ventricles of the
    heart: _____

14. pertaining to the armpit:

    _____

15. pertaining to around the ventricles:

    _____

16. hardening of the arteries:

    _____

17. enlargement of blood vessels:

    _____

18. resembling the ear:

    _____

19. incision into the abdomen:

    _____

20. stoppage of the flow of blood:

    _____

Identifying Abdominal Quadrants and Regions

Identify the correct term for each abdominal region shown on the image here.

1. _____

2. _____

3. _____

4. _____

5. _____

6. _____

7. _____

8. _____

9. _____

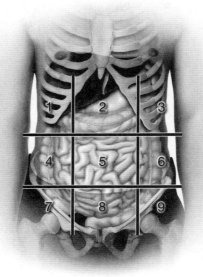

© Body Scientific International

Identify the correct term for each abdominal quadrant shown on the image here.

10. _____

11. _____

12. _____

13. _____

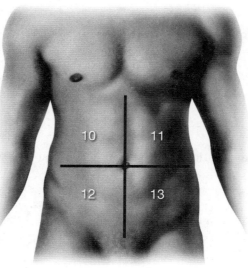

© Body Scientific International

Answer the following questions.

14. Which vital organs are located in the left upper quadrant?

_____

15. How do healthcare providers use the abdominal regions and quadrants to diagnose health issues?

_____

_____

_____

Name _____   Date _____

Understanding Directional Terms

Match each of the following definitions with the correct directional term. You will not use all of the terms.

A. abduction   G. extension   M. proximal
B. adduction   H. flexion   N. sagittal plane
C. coronal plane   I. inferior   O. superficial
D. deep   J. lateral   P. superior
E. distal   K. medial   Q. transverse plane
F. dorsal   L. midsagittal plane R. ventral

_____ 1. divides the body evenly into left and right sides

_____ 2. the anterior side of the body

_____ 3. the farthest area from the point of attachment

_____ 4. pertaining to the midline of the body

_____ 5. bending a limb to decrease the joint angle

_____ 6. movement of a limb away from the body

_____ 7. divides the body into upper and lower parts

_____ 8. closer to the feet

_____ 9. farther away from the surface of the body

_____ 10. closer to the point of attachment

_____ 11. divides the body into front and back halves

_____ 12. the back side of the body

_____ 13. closer to the surface of the body

_____ 14. straightening a limb to increase the joint angle

_____ 15. movement of a limb toward the body

Identifying Body Positions

Identify each body position shown here.

1.

Position: _____

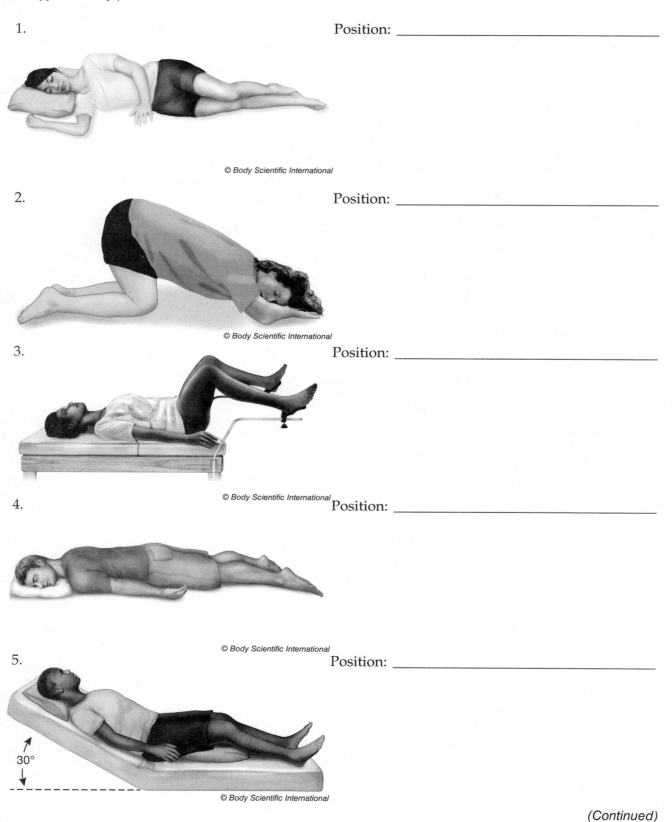

© Body Scientific International

2.

Position: _____

© Body Scientific International

3.

Position: _____

© Body Scientific International

4.

Position: _____

© Body Scientific International

5.

Position: _____

30°

© Body Scientific International

(Continued)

6.   Position: _____

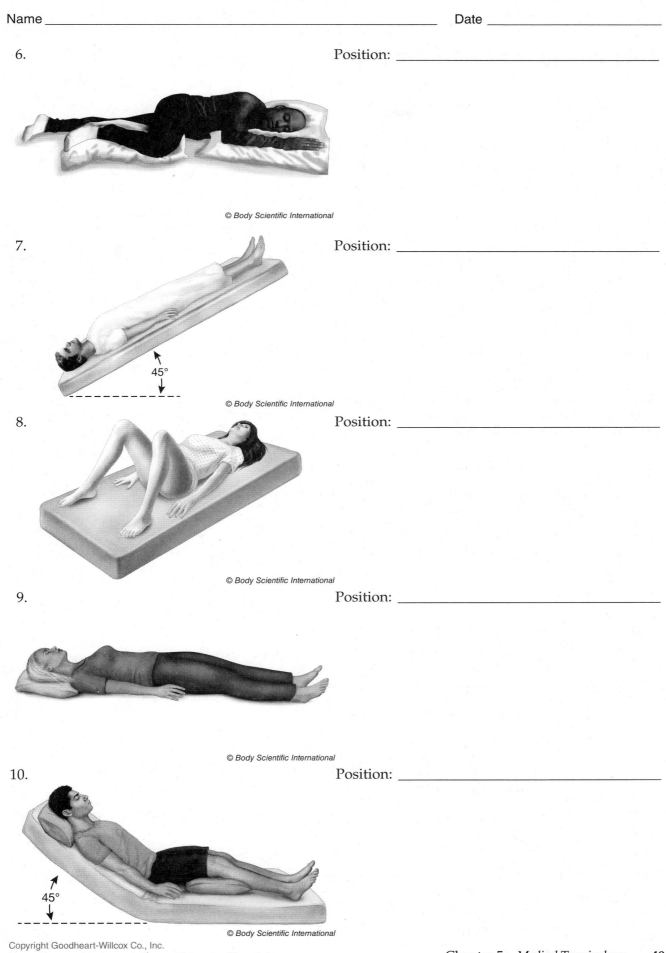

© Body Scientific International

7.   Position: _____

45°

© Body Scientific International

8.   Position: _____

© Body Scientific International

9.   Position: _____

© Body Scientific International

10.   Position: _____

45°

© Body Scientific International

Abbreviations and Acronyms

Define each of the following abbreviations and acronyms.

1. DOB: _____

2. CBC: _____

3. TIA: _____

4. MI: _____

5. Hgb: _____

6. OR: _____

7. wt: _____

8. ENT: _____

9. BS: _____

10. COPD: _____

11. Dx: _____

12. TPR: _____

13. NPO: _____

14. p/o: _____

15. UA: _____

16. FUO: _____

17. CA: _____

Each of the following items is a chart entry made by a healthcare professional to document patient care. Rewrite each statement without using abbreviations or acronyms. Look up the meaning of any abbreviations or acronyms that are not listed in the chapter.

18. Pt c/o elevated temp x3 days

VS: T—101.8; P—84; R—16; BP—132/80; wt—184 lbs, ht—64 inches

_____

_____

_____

_____

19. 8 y/o female patient c/o ear pain

HEENT exam: RT ear inflamed c̄ serous drainage; otherwise normal

_____

_____

_____

_____

20. 26 y/o male pt c/o intermittent chest pain

UA and CBC normal; AP & lat chest X-rays normal; ordered nuclear stress test to R/O CAD

_____

_____

_____

_____

Chapter 6

Anatomy and Physiology

Name _____ Date _____

Learning Anatomy and Physiology Terminology

Use the terms listed here to fill in the blanks in the following statements.

anatomy	central nervous system (CNS)	endocrine	joint
antibody		exocrine	ligaments
antigen	cytoplasm	formed elements	lymph
bone marrow	deoxyribonucleic acid (DNA)	homeostasis	lymphocyte
cell membrane		hormones	
chromosomes	differentiation	immunity	

1. The 23 pairs of threadlike structures that are found in the nucleus of most living cells and which carry important genetic information are known as _____.

2. Also known as an *articulation*, a(n) _____ is the physical point of connection between two bones.

3. Through the process of _____, cells of the body vary according to their specific function.

4. The study of the structure of the body is known as _____.

5. _____ glands secrete chemical substances called *hormones* to regulate body functions.

6. The selectively permeable outer layer of a cell that holds the cell together is called the

   _____.

7. The _____ is a transparent, gel-like substance found within the cell that houses all of the microscopic functioning units of the cell.

8. _____ is shaped like a twisting ladder, composed of chemical base pairs, and is part of all living cells.

9. _____ is a self-regulating process by which all biological functions in the body work together to maintain the stability of the organism.

(Continued)

10. The tough, white bands of fibrous tissue that connect bone to bone are known as

    _____.

11. The _____ includes the brain and spinal cord.

12. Chemical substances secreted by the endocrine glands to regulate different functions of the body

    are known as _____.

13. _____ glands contain ducts, allowing them to secrete their enzymes

    directly at the site of action.

14. The ability of the body to resist pathogens is called _____.

15. _____ is a colorless fluid from the body's tissues that carries white blood

    cells, collects and transports bacteria to the lymph nodes for destruction, and carries fats from the

    digestive system.

16. Any foreign substance from outside or inside the body that causes the immune system to pro-

    duce antibodies is known as a(n) _____.

17. A(n) _____ is a white blood cell that destroys pathogenic microorganisms.

18. A(n) _____ is a protein produced by the immune system that circulates in

    the plasma in response to the presence of foreign antigens.

19. The solid cellular components of blood, including red blood cells, white blood cells, and platelets,

    are called the _____.

20. _____ is the soft, flexible, spongy, blood-forming tissue found inside

    bones.

Identifying Parts of a Cell

In today's world, when the word cell *is used, the first thing that might come to mind is your phone. However, in reference to anatomy and physiology, the word* cell *is one of the most important words used to discuss the human body. Without our approximately five trillion* cells, *we would have no tissues, organs, or body systems. The cell is considered the basic unit of life in a living organism. Label the different parts of the cell shown in the image below.*

cell membrane	Golgi apparatus	peroxisome	smooth endoplasmic reticulum
centrosome	lysosome	ribosomes	
cytoplasm	mitochondrion	rough endoplasmic reticulum	
cytoskeleton	nucleus		

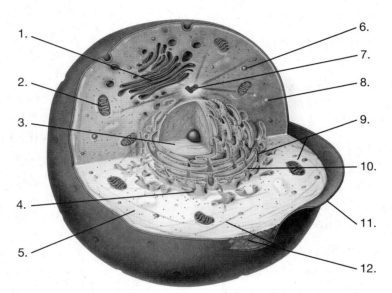

© *Body Scientific International*

1. _____

2. _____

3. _____

4. _____

5. _____

6. _____

7. _____

8. _____

9. _____

10. _____

11. _____

12. _____

Anatomy and Physiology Matching

Match each of the following definitions with the correct term. You will not use all of the terms.

_____ 1. groups of cells that work together to accomplish a task

_____ 2. part of the formed elements that fight infection in the body

_____ 3. the act of supplying oxygen to the cells and removing carbon dioxide from the body

_____ 4. the "brain" of the cell, which directs all cellular activities and contains genetic information

_____ 5. a process or stage of life that indicates sexual reproduction is possible

_____ 6. the collective term for nerves that lie outside the CNS and transmit information from the CNS to all parts of the body

_____ 7. cells in the body that evolve into specific cells in a particular organ system

_____ 8. part of the formed elements that contain hemoglobin, which carries oxygen and carbon dioxide to and from the body's cells

_____ 9. the process in which white blood cells surround, ingest, and destroy a foreign invader

_____ 10. the study of the function of the body

_____ 11. part of the formed elements that play an important role in blood clotting

_____ 12. the chemical processes occurring within a living organism, which maintain life

_____ 13. a system for measuring a substance's level of acidity or alkalinity

_____ 14. the study of the structure of the body

_____ 15. an infection transferred from one person to another through sexual contact

A. anatomy
B. metabolism
C. nucleus
D. organs
E. peripheral nervous system
F. pH scale
G. phagocytosis
H. physiology
I. plasma
J. platelets
K. puberty
L. red blood cells
M. respiration
N. sexually transmitted infection
O. stem cells
P. tendons
Q. tissues
R. white blood cells

Date _____

How Well Do You Know Your Glands?

Match each of the following endocrine glands with the function it performs.

_____ 1. regulates and aids in the secretion of essential hormones

_____ 2. produces thyroxine and triiodothyronine to regulate the metabolism of proteins, carbohydrates, and fats

_____ 3. stimulates or inhibits pituitary secretions and integrates responses from the nervous system

_____ 4. releases melatonin to control sleep

_____ 5. contains the islets of Langerhans, which secrete glucagon and insulin

_____ 6. affects metabolism and growth

_____ 7. stimulates the production of T and B cells to aid in the immune response

_____ 8. contribute to the development of female sex characteristics

_____ 9. maintain blood calcium levels

_____ 10. produce testosterone in males

A. pancreas
B. thyroid gland
C. parathyroid glands
D. adrenal gland
E. ovaries
F. pituitary gland
G. testes
H. pineal gland
I. thymus gland
J. hypothalamus

Body System Bingo

Regular Game Rules

Your teacher will announce five body systems to be used in the game. Write those body systems in the top row of boxes on the bingo card shown here. Then determine five organs that can be found in each of those body systems. Write one organ in each box under the corresponding body system. Once every student has a completed bingo card, your teacher will name an organ from one of the body systems. If you have that organ on your card, mark the appropriate box in some way. Your teacher will continue to name organs, and you will continue to mark boxes if he or she calls an organ that you have listed. Once a student has five boxes marked in a row (either across, up and down, or diagonally), he or she will call out "bingo," or any other word the teacher finds appropriate. That student is the winner.

Advanced Game Rules

Your teacher will announce five body systems to be used in the game. Write those body systems in the top row of boxes on the bingo card shown here. Then determine five organs that can be found in each of those body systems. Write one organ in each box under the corresponding body system. Once every student has a completed bingo card, your teacher will name the function of an organ. If you have the organ associated with that function listed on your bingo card, mark the appropriate box. Your teacher will continue to name the functions of organs, and you will continue to mark boxes if you have listed the organs that match those functions. Once a student has five boxes marked in a row (either across, up and down, or diagonally), he or she will call out "bingo," or any other word the teacher finds appropriate. That student is the winner.

BODY SYSTEM:	BODY SYSTEM:	BODY SYSTEM:	BODY SYSTEM:	BODY SYSTEM:
ORGAN:	ORGAN:	ORGAN:	ORGAN:	ORGAN:
ORGAN:	ORGAN:	ORGAN:	ORGAN:	ORGAN:
ORGAN:	ORGAN:	ORGAN:	ORGAN:	ORGAN:
ORGAN:	ORGAN:	ORGAN:	ORGAN:	ORGAN:
ORGAN:	ORGAN:	ORGAN:	ORGAN:	ORGAN:

Labeling the Integumentary System

Using the word bank provided here, label the different components of the skin shown in the image below.

artery   lipocytes   sweat gland
dermis   nerve fibers   sweat gland duct
epidermis   pore of sweat gland duct   tactile corpuscle
hair   sebaceous gland   vein
hair follicle   subcutaneous

© Body Scientific International

1. _____   8. _____
2. _____   9. _____
3. _____   10. _____
4. _____   11. _____
5. _____   12. _____
6. _____   13. _____
7. _____   14. _____

Name _____ Date _____

Labeling the Skeletal System

Using the word bank provided here, label the different bones of the skeleton shown in the image below. You may use some terms in the word bank more than once.

calcaneus	cranium	metacarpals	ribs	tarsals
carpals	facial bones	metatarsals	sacrum	thoracic cage
clavicle	femur	patella	scapula	tibia
coccyx	fibula	phalanges	skull	ulna
coxal bone	humerus	radius	sternum	vertebral column

1. _____

2. _____

3. _____

4. _____

5. _____

6. _____

7. _____

8. _____

9. _____

10. _____

11. _____

12. _____

13. _____

14. _____

15. _____

16. _____

17. _____

18. _____

19. _____

20. _____

21. _____

22. _____

23. _____

24. _____

25. _____

26. _____

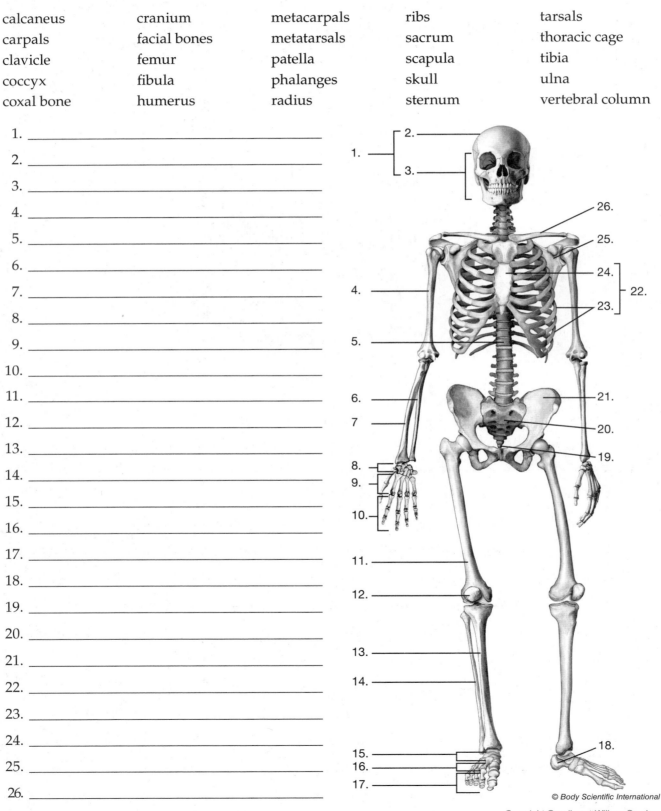

© Body Scientific International

Name _____ Date _____

Labeling the Muscular System

Using the word bank provided here, label the different muscles shown in the image below.

abdominal   biceps femoris   gastrocnemius   latissimus dorsi   sartorius
   muscles   deltoid   gluteus maximus   pectoralis major   trapezius
Achilles tendon   frontalis   gluteus medius   rectus femoris   triceps brachii
biceps brachii

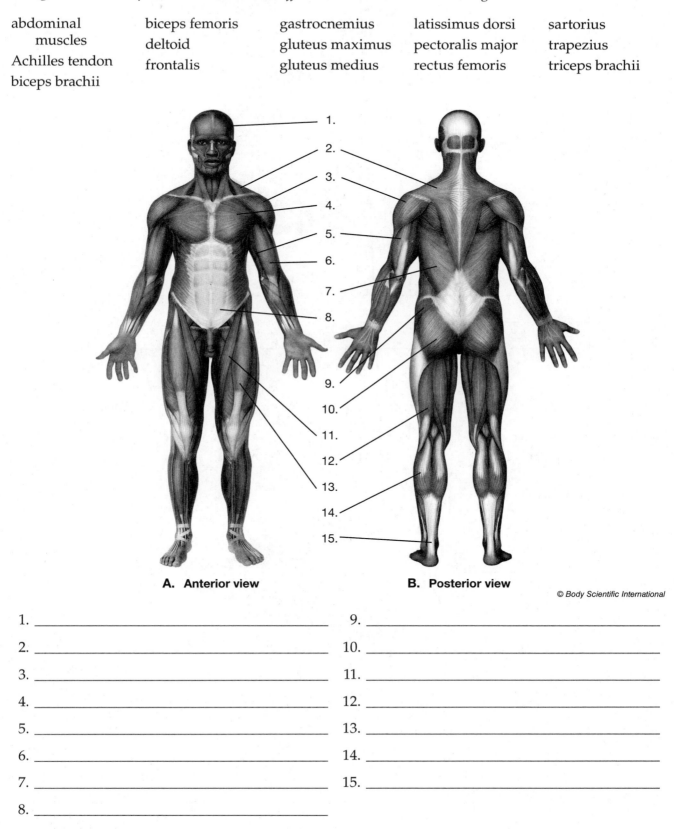

A. Anterior view   **B. Posterior view**

© Body Scientific International

1. _____   9. _____

2. _____   10. _____

3. _____   11. _____

4. _____   12. _____

5. _____   13. _____

6. _____   14. _____

7. _____   15. _____

8. _____

Name _____ Date _____

Labeling the Nervous and Sensory Systems

Using the word bank provided here, label the different areas of the brain shown in the image below.

brainstem   cerebrum   midbrain   spinal cord
cerebellum   medulla oblongata pons

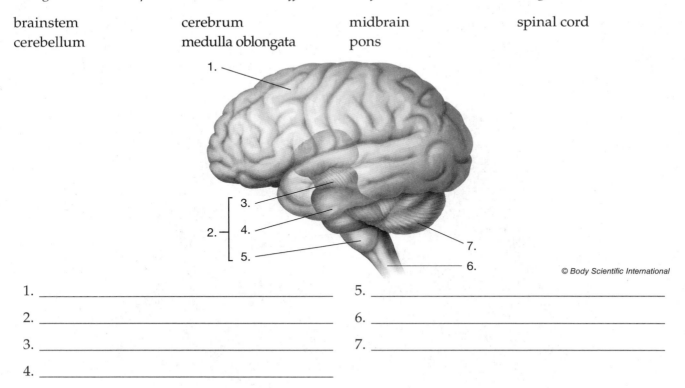

© Body Scientific International

1. _____   5. _____

2. _____   6. _____

3. _____   7. _____

4. _____

Using the word bank provided here, label the different parts of the eye shown in the image below.

cornea   eyelashes   iris   orbital muscles   retina
eye socket   eyelid   optic nerve   pupil   sclera

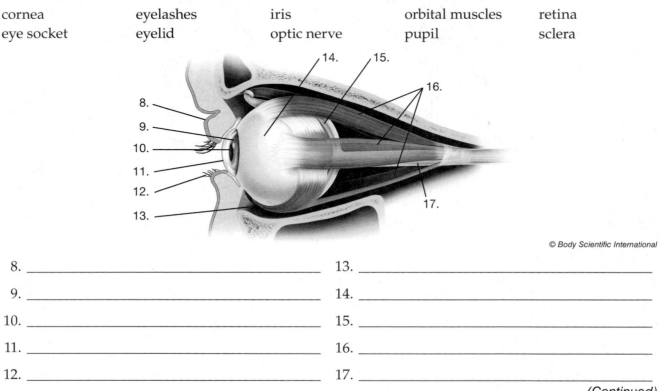

© Body Scientific International

8. _____   13. _____

9. _____   14. _____

10. _____   15. _____

11. _____   16. _____

12. _____   17. _____

(Continued)

Name _____   Date _____

Using the word bank provided here, label the different parts of the ear shown in the image below.

anvil   external auditory canal   ossicles   semicircular canals
auricle   hammer   outer ear   stirrup
cochlea   inner ear   oval window   tympanic membrane
Eustachian tube   middle ear   round window   vestibulocochlear
                                                                          nerve

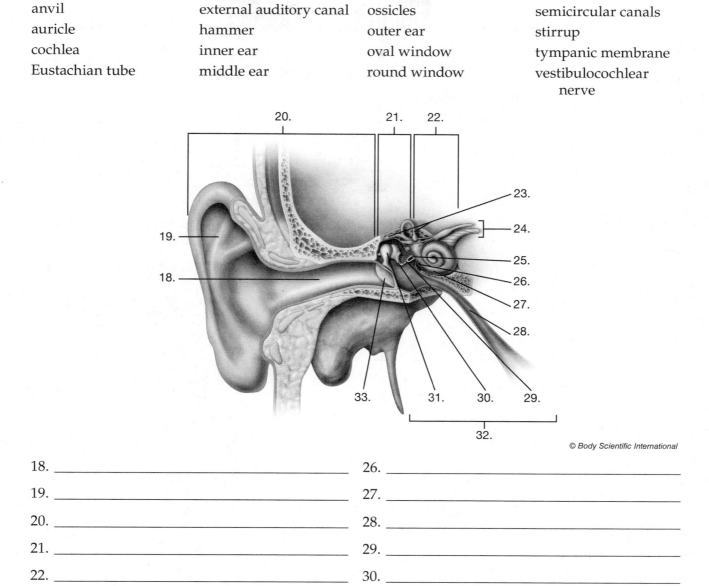

© Body Scientific International

18. _____   26. _____
19. _____   27. _____
20. _____   28. _____
21. _____   29. _____
22. _____   30. _____
23. _____   31. _____
24. _____   32. _____
25. _____   33. _____

Name _____   Date _____

Labeling the Endocrine System

Using the word bank provided here, label the different glands of the endocrine system shown in the image below.

adrenal glands   pancreas   pituitary gland   thyroid gland
hypothalamus   parathyroid gland   testis
ovary   pineal gland   thymus gland

1. _____

2. _____

3. _____

4. _____

5. _____

6. _____

7. _____

8. _____

9. _____

10. _____

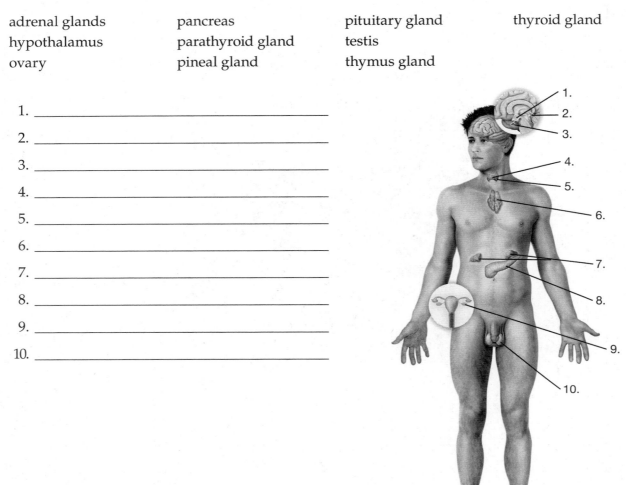

© Body Scientific International

Labeling the Respiratory System

Using the word bank provided here, label the different parts of the respiratory system shown in the image below. You may use some terms in the word bank more than once.

alveoli	diaphragm	pharynx	trachea
bronchi	larynx	pulmonary arteriole	
bronchiole	left lung	pulmonary venule	
capillaries	nose	right lung	

© Body Scientific International

1. _____
2. _____
3. _____
4. _____
5. _____
6. _____
7. _____

8. _____
9. _____
10. _____
11. _____
12. _____
13. _____
14. _____

Labeling the Cardiovascular System

Using the word bank provided here, label the different parts of the heart shown in the image below.

aortic arch
aortic valve
chordae tendineae
descending aorta
endocardium
inferior vena cava

left atrium
left pulmonary artery
   to left lung
left pulmonary veins
left ventricle
mitral valve
myocardium

papillary muscles
pericardium
pulmonary trunk
pulmonary valve
right atrium
right pulmonary artery
   to right lung

right pulmonary veins
right ventricle
septum
superior vena cava
tricuspid valve

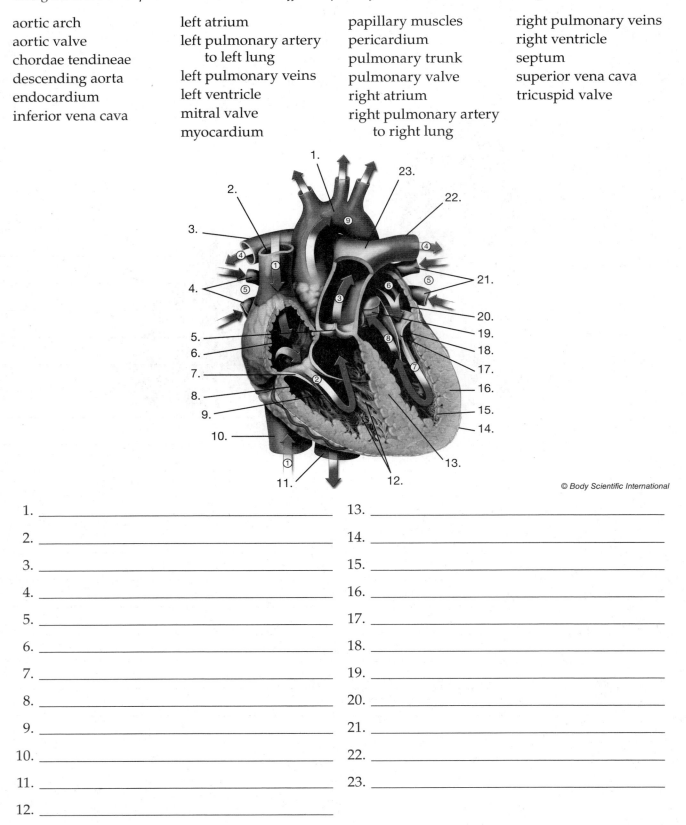

© Body Scientific International

1. _____
2. _____
3. _____
4. _____
5. _____
6. _____
7. _____
8. _____
9. _____
10. _____
11. _____
12. _____

13. _____
14. _____
15. _____
16. _____
17. _____
18. _____
19. _____
20. _____
21. _____
22. _____
23. _____

Labeling the Gastrointestinal System

Using the word bank provided here, label the different parts of the gastrointestinal system shown in the image below.

anus	liver	pharynx	stomach
esophagus	mouth	rectum	sublingual
gallbladder	pancreas	salivary glands	submandibular
large intestine	parotid	small intestine	

1. _____

2. _____

3. _____

4. _____

5. _____

6. _____

7. _____

8. _____

9. _____

10. _____

11. _____

12. _____

13. _____

14. _____

15. _____

© Body Scientific International

Name _____   Date _____

Labeling the Urinary System

Using the word bank provided here, label the different parts of the kidney shown in the image below.

renal capsule   renal cortex   renal pelvis   ureter
renal column   renal medulla   renal pyramid

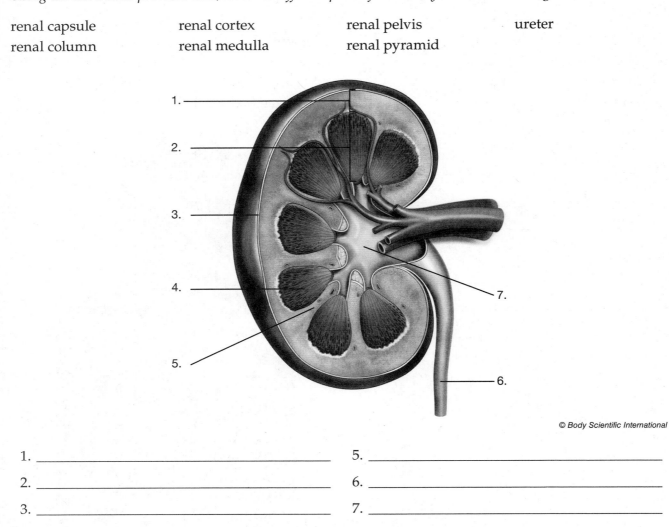

© Body Scientific International

1. _____   5. _____
2. _____   6. _____
3. _____   7. _____
4. _____

Chapter 7

Disease

Name _____ Date _____

Classifying Diseases and Disorders

Classify each disease, disorder, or injury according to its cause. Write the letter of the correct classification in the space provided. Classifications may be used more than once.

_____ 1. sickle cell anemia

_____ 2. hepatitis C

_____ 3. broken leg

_____ 4. influenza

_____ 5. Down syndrome

_____ 6. black lung disease

_____ 7. obesity

_____ 8. skin cancer

_____ 9. tetanus

_____ 10. cerebral palsy

_____ 11. Alzheimer's disease

_____ 12. rickets

_____ 13. osteoarthritis

_____ 14. fetal alcohol syndrome

_____ 15. silicosis

_____ 16. bulimia nervosa

_____ 17. measles

_____ 18. third-degree burn

A. congenital

B. degenerative

C. environmental

D. hereditary

E. infectious

F. nutritional

G. traumatic

Name _____   Date _____

Identifying Medical Specialties

Read each of the following descriptions of treatment and identify the medical specialist typically associated with the type of care or area of medicine described. Use a medical dictionary to look up any diseases or terms with which you are not familiar.

1. A 1-day-old baby is placed under an ultraviolet light to treat jaundice that developed due to a buildup of bilirubin in the body. _____

2. A 10-year-old boy has a cavity filled. _____

3. A 53-year-old woman undergoes a procedure to remove a squamous cell carcinoma from her left cheek. _____

4. A 6-year-old girl is given a prescription for an antibiotic after being diagnosed with chicken pox.

_____

5. A researcher publishes a study on the use of beta-blocker medications in heart disease patients.

_____

6. A woman's primary care provider sends her to this specialist for COPD treatment.

_____

7. A man is sent to the radiology department for an X-ray of his foot, which may be broken. The technologist doesn't see any fractures, but the films must be read by this specialist before the result is final. _____

8. A patient with post-traumatic stress disorder undergoes talk therapy. Her specialist also prescribes an antidepressant. _____

9. A woman who is four months pregnant has a checkup and an amniocentesis procedure.

_____

10. An 87-year-old man sees this specialist because he has been feeling very tired and having frequent headaches. _____

11. A 43-year-old business executive undergoes an endoscopy procedure to determine the cause of frequent abdominal pain and a burning sensation in his stomach. _____

12. A team of specialists is organized to study an outbreak of avian influenza in China.

_____

13. A 27-year-old man is diagnosed with hypertension, so he is referred to this specialist to discuss changes in his diet. _____

14. A 38-year-old patient undergoes surgery after falling and shattering his left forearm at his construction job. _____

15. A woman is referred to this specialist because she has had cystitis three times in the last year.

_____

Understanding Disease Terms

Match each of the following definitions with the correct disease-related term. You will not use all of the terms.

_____ 1. a subjective finding that is experienced by the patient

_____ 2. term that describes a long-lasting disease

_____ 3. term that describes a disease inherited through a person's genes

_____ 4. term that describes a disease that typically does not last long

_____ 5. a prediction of the probable outcome of a disease

_____ 6. the term for two or more coexisting diseases

_____ 7. an objective finding that can be seen upon observation

_____ 8. a disease that is prevalent in a particular group of people or a specific region

_____ 9. the number of deaths in a given population

_____ 10. term for a disease that is confined to a certain area of the body

_____ 11. a disease that affects an unusually large number of the population

_____ 12. term that describes a disease of unknown origin or cause

_____ 13. the act of determining the cause of a disease

_____ 14. a group of symptoms that indicate a disease, psychological disorder, or other abnormal condition

_____ 15. term that describes a condition present at birth

_____ 16. term for a disease that affects a large part or most of the body

A. acute
B. benign
C. chronic
D. comorbidity
E. congenital
F. diagnosis
G. endemic
H. epidemic
I. hereditary
J. idiopathic
K. localized
L. morbidity
M. mortality
N. pandemic
O. prognosis
P. sign
Q. symptom
R. syndrome
S. systemic

Name _____ Date _____

Biotechnology Issues

The field of biotechnology is not new. As early as 500 BCE, Chinese practitioners deliberately allowed soybean curds to become moldy. They then used these curds as an antibiotic (although the term had not yet been invented) to treat boils. More recently, biotechnology has been responsible for the introduction of vaccines, the discovery of cancer-causing viruses, and the hybridization of food plants, such as corn.

However, biotechnology has always been controversial. It has become more controversial in the last 50 years, as science and technology have advanced so far that ethical questions must be considered. This chapter describes some of the controversy surrounding cloning and stem cell research, but all types of genetic research, including many gene therapies, are also controversial.

Consider the current issues in biotechnology. Conduct research if necessary to find out exactly what the issues are. Choose one issue that interests you. Then use reputable sources to research both the pros and the cons of the issue. Record your findings in the table below. Then write a summary of your findings, including your conclusions about the issue. Be sure to back up your conclusions with solid research.

Biotechnology Issue:	
Pros (Why should this technology be approved or used? What are its benefits?)	**Cons** (Why should this technology be prevented? What are its drawbacks?)

Summary:

_____

_____

_____

_____

_____

Name _____   Date _____

Identifying Signs and Symptoms

Identify the signs and symptoms for each disease listed in the table below. You may need to conduct research to find the common symptoms for some of these diseases.

Disease	Signs and Symptoms
rheumatoid arthritis	
Alzheimer's disease	
coronary artery disease	
colorectal cancer	
COPD	
bronchitis	
diabetes	
influenza	
pneumonia	
kidney disease	

(Continued)

Review the symptoms you listed in the table. Then answer the following questions.

1. Why might it be difficult for medical professionals to diagnose a specific illness?

_____

_____

_____

_____

_____

2. What can medical professionals do to increase the accuracy of their diagnoses?

_____

_____

_____

_____

_____

3. In your opinion, why has healthcare reform emphasized the patient's role in maintaining his or her own health?

_____

_____

_____

_____

_____

_____

_____

_____

The Caregiver's Role

Many diseases have major consequences not only for the patient, but also for his or her family, friends, and especially the primary caregiver. Diseases and conditions such as Alzheimer's disease, stroke, cancer, and congestive heart failure sometimes require important lifestyle changes, which the patient may or may not be able to achieve without help.

The role of the caregiver in such cases has recently become a genuine medical focus. Physicians and other practitioners recognize that, without the caregiver, ongoing patient care becomes difficult unless the patient is institutionalized. Placing the patient in a nursing or rehabilitation facility is not always possible or desirable. However, when the patient remains in the home setting, the patient's primary caregiver faces many physical and psychological challenges. Many communities and organizations now exist to help support the caregiver, who in turn can provide the level of care the patient requires.

Choose one of the diseases mentioned in this chapter and conduct research to find out more about the support networks that exist for the caregivers of patients who have this disease. Record your findings here. Be prepared to share this information with your classmates and with people in your life who may care for someone suffering from this disease.

Disease researched: _____

Frequent needs of caregivers for patients who have this disease: _____

_____

_____

_____

_____

_____

Caregiver support organizations: _____

_____

_____

_____

_____

_____

_____

Types of support offered: _____

_____

_____

_____

_____

_____

Chapter 8

Health and Wellness

Name _____ Date _____

Understanding Health and Wellness Concepts

Use the terms listed here to fill in the blanks in the following statements.

addiction	depression	self-esteem
aerobic exercise	emotional intelligence	stress
anorexia nervosa	endorphins	substance abuse
bipolar disorder	euphoria	suicide
body image	health literacy	suicide cluster
bulimia nervosa	holistic health	suicide contagion
complementary and alternative medicine	meditation	

1. The term _____ refers to a broad variety of practices that include techniques designed to promote relaxation and harmony with your environment.

2. The term _____ describes the use of illegal drugs or alcohol, or the misuse of prescription medication.

3. A person's _____ includes thoughts and feelings about how he or she looks.

4. Hormones secreted within the brain during exercise, which reduce the sensation of pain or stress, are known as _____.

5. _____ is the measure of one's ability to be aware of, control, and express one's emotions and to maintain successful interpersonal relations.

6. Intentionally ending one's life is known as _____.

7. _____ is a mental disorder characterized by alternating periods of euphoria and depression.

8. An individual's _____ is defined by his or her ability to obtain, communicate, and understand basic health information and services, allowing him or her to make appropriate health decisions.

(Continued)

9. Physical activities such as running or swimming are called _____, meaning that they require the heart to deliver oxygenated blood to working muscles.

10. A(n) _____ occurs when multiple suicides take place within a community during a relatively short period of time.

11. Your _____ is shaped by what you think and feel about yourself.

12. The eating disorder known as _____ is characterized by bingeing and purging.

13. _____ is a wellness approach that advocates treating a patient's physical, emotional, mental, and spiritual health.

14. The emotional and mental condition in which a person experiences intense feelings of well-being, happiness, and excitement is called _____.

15. The body's physical, mental, and emotional response to change, trauma, or challenging situations is called _____.

16. The physical and psychological need for a habit-forming substance, such as drugs or alcohol, or an activity, such as shopping, is known as a(n) _____.

17. _____ is a mood disorder characterized by feelings of hopelessness, worthlessness, or a general disinterest in daily life.

18. Health practices used in place of or in conjunction with traditional Western medicine are known as _____, or integrative health.

19. The term _____ describes the copying of suicide attempts after hearing about another person's suicide.

20. _____ is an eating disorder characterized by low weight, fear of gaining weight, and food restrictions.

Health and Wellness Discussion Questions

Answer the following questions.

1. Name six main areas you should focus on to keep the physical body healthy.

   _____

   _____

   _____

   _____

   _____

   _____

2. List eight habits you can incorporate into your life to maintain a healthy diet.

   _____

   _____

   _____

   _____

   _____

   _____

   _____

   _____

   _____

   _____

3. What are the benefits of establishing a regular plan for exercise?

   _____

   _____

   _____

   _____

   _____

   _____

4. How much sleep should most teenagers get every night?

   _____

(Continued)

Name _____ Date _____

5. List five harmful or negative effects of addiction and substance abuse.

_____

_____

_____

_____

_____

6. Why is addiction and substance abuse especially harmful for those working in healthcare?

_____

_____

_____

_____

7. Define *social health* in your own words. What are the benefits of having good social health?

_____

_____

_____

_____

8. Describe the type A, type B, and type C personalities. Which of the three types best describes your own personality?

_____

_____

_____

_____

_____

9. List five strategies for working through stress and achieving a positive outcome.

_____

_____

_____

_____

_____

10. List five complementary and alternative medicine practices used today.

_____

_____

_____

Complementary and Alternative Medicine

Match the following descriptions with the correct complementary and alternative medicine practice.

A. hypnotherapy   C. aromatherapy   E. naturopathy   G. homeopathy
B. yoga   D. acupuncture   F. reflexology   H. Reiki

_____ 1. This therapy includes applying pressure to specific points on the foot so energy is directed toward the affected body part. It is an ancient art based on the concept that the body is divided into 10 zones that run from the head to the toes, and that illness or disease of the body causes deposits of calcium or acids in the corresponding part of the foot. This therapy is used to promote healing and relaxation; improve circulation; and treat asthma, sinus infections, IBS, kidney stones, and constipation.

_____ 2. This therapy includes the use of selected fragrances and oils from roots, bark, plants, and flowers to relieve muscle tension, tension headaches, or backaches. It is also used to help lower blood pressure and create a soothing effect in the body.

_____ 3. This ancient Japanese and Tibetan art is based on the idea that disease causes an imbalance in the body's energy field. It is also known as the *healing touch* because gentle hand pressure is applied to the body's energy centers, known as *chakras*, to harness and balance the life energy force. It is also believed to help clear blockages in the body and stimulate healing.

_____ 4. This practice includes all natural therapies, such as special diets, lifestyle changes, and supportive approaches to promote healing and treat illness, while avoiding the use of medicines and surgery.

_____ 5. This practice induces a trance-like state so a person is receptive to suggestion. It is used to encourage desired behavior changes, such as losing weight or stopping smoking.

_____ 6. This ancient Chinese therapy involves the insertion of very thin needles into specific points along the pathways of the body to stimulate and balance the flow of energy, referred to as *qi*. This belief is based on the concept that illness and pain occur when the *qi* is blocked.

_____ 7. This practice uses very small doses of drugs made from natural substances to produce symptoms of a disease being treated. It is based on the belief that these natural substances will stimulate the immune system to heal the body.

_____ 8. This Hindu discipline uses concentration, specific positions, and ancient ritual movements to maintain the balance and flow of life energy. It is used to increase spiritual enlightenment and well-being and to develop an awareness of the body to improve coordination, relieve stress, and improve muscle tone.

Name_____ Date _____

Personal Reflection Exercise

Once you have finished studying this chapter, consider the health and wellness strategies you have learned. Choose the 10 strategies that you feel will help your personal health and wellness and record them here. In addition, describe how and when you plan to implement these practices.

_____

_____

_____

_____

_____

_____

_____

_____

_____

_____

_____

_____

_____

_____

_____

_____

_____

_____

_____

_____

_____

_____

_____

_____

Chapter 9

Lifespan Development

Name _____ Date _____

Maslow's Hierarchy

Fill in each level of Maslow's hierarchy of human needs on the image below. Then, in the bubble attached to each level, list two ways in which that need can be met.

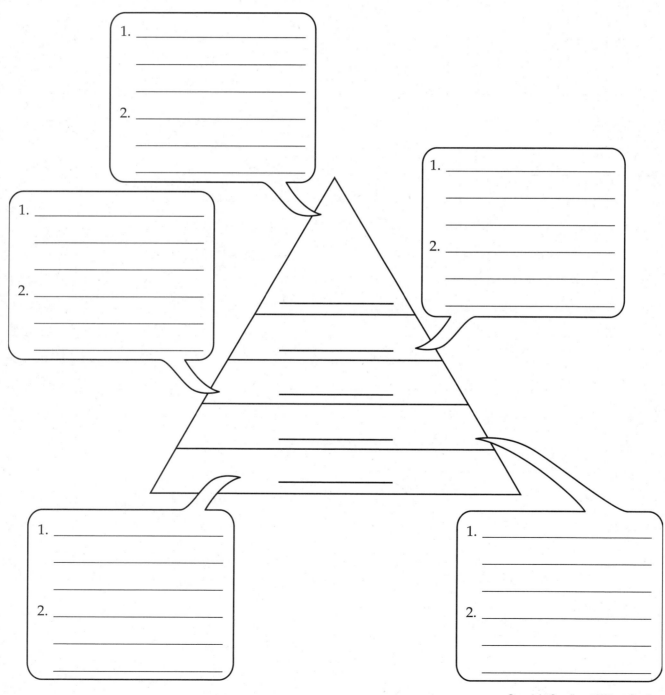

Identifying the Stages of Life

List the age range associated with each life stage listed below. Then match each of the following developments or characteristics with the life stage in which it occurs. You may use each life stage more than once.

A. prenatal: _____

B. infancy: _____

C. early childhood: _____

D. middle childhood: _____

E. late childhood: _____

F. adolescence: _____

G. early adulthood: _____

H. middle adulthood: _____

I. late adulthood: _____

_____ 1. Individuals must be monitored constantly to ensure their safety as they begin to walk and are able to open cabinets.

_____ 2. Females begin to menstruate.

_____ 3. Wrinkles and age spots appear, and osteoporosis poses a risk of broken bones.

_____ 4. The three parts of this life stage are called *trimesters*.

_____ 5. Hormone production slows in men.

_____ 6. Rooting and startle reflexes are present.

_____ 7. Individuals may feel depressed as they face the reality of their eventual death.

_____ 8. Coordination and muscle development are at their peak.

_____ 9. Sexual maturation and changes in body functions occur.

_____ 10. Toilet training occurs.

_____ 11. Although bonding can occur throughout a person's life span, it is particularly important in this stage.

_____ 12. Team sports are encouraged because they help improve motor skills and social skills.

_____ 13. Women experience menopause.

_____ 14. Individuals begin to better understand abstract concepts such as honesty and loyalty.

_____ 15. In Western societies, a midlife crisis may occur during this stage.

Analyzing Childhood Obesity

The percentage of children and adolescents who are obese is becoming alarmingly high. Childhood obesity can have lifelong effects, potentially contributing to problems with almost every body system. Use reliable sources to research this growing problem. Then answer the following questions.

1. What percentage of children and adolescents is considered obese?

   _____

2. What are the major causes of childhood obesity?

   _____

   _____

   _____

   _____

   _____

3. What are the common consequences of childhood obesity?

   _____

   _____

   _____

   _____

   _____

4. What techniques are recommended to help prevent childhood obesity?

   _____

   _____

   _____

   _____

   _____

5. List some possible solutions to the problem of childhood obesity.

   _____

   _____

   _____

   _____

   _____

   _____

Recognizing Stages of Grief

Being able to identify when people are grieving, and the stage of grief they are experiencing, is an important skill for healthcare workers, particularly for those who work in gerontology practices. Knowing the stage of grief a patient is experiencing enables the healthcare worker to understand and respond to the patient's needs appropriately. Listed below are several statements made by patients who know that they are dying or that someone close to them is dying. Match each of these statements with the correct stage of grief. You may use each stage of grief more than once.

A. denial
B. anger
C. bargaining
D. depression
E. acceptance

_____ 1. "No, thanks, I don't want to go to lunch. I'm just not hungry today."

_____ 2. "I think I'm going now. Will you stay here and hold my hand while it happens?"

_____ 3. "The doctor says I have stomach cancer, but he doesn't know what he's talking about. Anyone can see that I have a healthy tummy!"

_____ 4. "Doctor, I know you believe my daughter is dying, but if you can save her, I'll pay double—even triple!—your usual fee."

_____ 5. "I've tried all my life to take good care of my body. I don't drink, smoke, or use any kind of drug. Now look what my body is doing to me! They say I have liver cancer! Stupid liver!"

_____ 6. "Yes, the oncologist says I have only three months to live. But that's what they told my cousin Emily four years ago, and she's still with us. I don't think anyone knows for sure, and I certainly don't feel like I'm dying!"

_____ 7. "Well, I've lived a good life. If my time has come, then I'm ready to go."

_____ 8. "Don't you touch my son with that blood pressure cuff! Can't you see he's already in such pain? Why don't you go pick on someone else?"

_____ 9. "You ask why I am crying? Why shouldn't I cry? It's about the only thing I can do, now that I'm too weak to stand or even hold a book."

_____ 10. "Now, honey, don't cry for me. I've lived a long time, and I think I made some small difference in the world. You go on, now, and make your mark. You have your whole life ahead of you."

Identifying Genetic Disorders

Match each genetic disorder with its effects. Then describe each disorder's cause and treatment options in the space provided.

A. cystic fibrosis
B. Down syndrome
C. fragile X syndrome
D. Huntington's disease
E. phenylketonuria
F. sickle cell anemia
G. spina bifida
H. Tay-Sachs disease

_____ 1. cognitive and physical deterioration, frequently resulting in early death

Cause: _____

_____

Treatment options: _____

_____

_____ 2. loss of memory, ability to rationalize, and some physical control, leading to depression and often death from complications

Cause: _____

_____

Treatment options: _____

_____

_____ 3. respiratory, digestive, and reproductive issues, with effects ranging from mild to severe

Cause: _____

_____

Treatment options: _____

_____

_____ 4. may have no effect or result in either chronic illness or early death

Cause: _____

_____

Treatment options: _____

_____

(Continued)

_____   5. non-uniform effects that include severe cognitive disability and delayed language development

Cause: _____

_____

Treatment options: _____

_____

_____   6. fluid buildup in the skull and partial to complete paralysis

Cause: _____

_____

Treatment options: _____

_____

_____   7. permanent internal damage and cognitive disability, if undetected

Cause: _____

_____

Treatment options: _____

_____

_____   8. effects range from short attention span to a learning disability to a severe cognitive disability

Cause: _____

_____

Treatment options: _____

_____

Life Stages around the World

It is well known that culture and society play important roles in human growth and development. These factors may affect physical characteristics, psychological and emotional development, and even the period of time included in each life stage. Choose a culture or society that is different from your own. Then choose one life stage on which to focus. Conduct research to discover the age range included in that life stage in your chosen culture or society, as well as the stage's characteristics in that culture or society. How is the life stage different from the same one in your community? Use the space below to take notes as you research. Then create an outline for a two-minute oral presentation. Be prepared to present your work to the class.

Notes:

_____

_____

_____

_____

_____

_____

_____

_____

_____

_____

_____

_____

_____

_____

_____

_____

_____

_____

_____

_____

_____

_____

(Continued)

Name _____ Date _____

Outline:

I. _____

_____

   A. _____

_____

   B. _____

_____

   C. _____

_____

II. _____

_____

   A. _____

_____

   B. _____

_____

   C. _____

_____

III. _____

_____

   A. _____

_____

   B. _____

_____

   C. _____

_____

Chapter 10

Healthcare Technology

Name _____ Date _____

Healthcare Technology Matching

Match each of the following definitions with the correct term related to healthcare technology. You will not use all of the terms.

_____ 1. an artificial replacement for a missing body part, such as a limb, an eye, a tooth, a hip, or a knee

_____ 2. the manipulation of genetic materials to eliminate undesirable traits or ensure desirable traits

_____ 3. prescription drugs that are produced as a result of biotechnology

_____ 4. legislation passed in 2009 to improve healthcare through increased use of health information technology

_____ 5. the use of learning machines and tools to show what a medical emergency looks like or how a healthcare procedure is performed

_____ 6. a mobile computer used to access and enter patient information around a healthcare facility

_____ 7. reports used during a shift change, or a change in the level of patient care, to explain a patient's status

_____ 8. the creation of an organism that is an exact genetic copy of another with identical DNA to its parent

_____ 9. a computerized record that contains information from a single medical practice or a single stay in one healthcare facility

_____ 10. field of medicine in which communication and information technologies are used to provide patients with medical care at remote locations

A. biopharmaceuticals
B. biotechnology
C. cloning
D. computer on wheels (COW)
E. electronic medical record (EMR)
F. genetic engineering
G. handoff reports
H. healthcare simulation
I. HITECH Act
J. prosthesis
K. telemedicine

Healthcare Technology Word Search

Search the grid of letters below for the terms listed in the word bank.

cloning	EMR	MRI	tablet
COW	handoff	PET	telemedicine
CT	HIPAA	prosthesis	X-ray
diagnosis	HITECH	record	
EHR	laser	robotics	

```
H O E F N T A P M R L A Q T B Y K U
N W N I X C E V I R E S A L Q C O Q
R Z R E M O A E R N J B P A E V K A
I H O S R C N H Q K L E I X P W U A
N U E S M T O R B E C I L E I R M P
A N P E D J H O T C I K W C Y I A I
O X F R O N A C O G L W B S A K X H
M R L O Y B N L R C L O N I N G C U
Q A C N P A D N I R E N O L T N Q T
M Y L V D R O C E R U M V E R V S E
J E X I N P F B Y L Q V N N L E C B
Z N P T N I F E O S N I Q V O D I S
B I L S Y N V P Z V C O M E J O T B
D I A G N O S I S I N E S O M W O L
B E I K S N A T D O L C E U S N B P
P O N A L R O E C M E A J W V D O F
H I N A P A M M U Q A O L N R B R V
B I P P A E L Q B T X B W P E V I N
L E C I L S H I L P E N G O K L A O
N P E E P R O S T H E S I S C L B G
I U T C L R E X A B Z T I K R N W C
M U R S O M M R C R B I E J Y F W D
H E H I T E C H N L U R X P M T G H
```

Healthcare Technology Discussion Questions

Answer the following questions.

1. List 10 healthcare office duties for which computers can be used.

_____

_____

_____

_____

_____

2. Describe what a typical hospital visit would be like without computers.

_____

_____

_____

_____

3. What is HIPAA? Why was HIPAA enacted?

_____

_____

_____

_____

4. What are handoff reports and why are they important?

_____

_____

_____

_____

5. Why is confidentiality especially important in healthcare?

_____

_____

_____

6. What does *EHR* stand for? What are the benefits of using an EHR?

_____

_____

_____

_____

(Continued)

7. What is the difference between an EHR and an EMR?

_____

_____

_____

8. What are the advantages of telemedicine?

_____

_____

_____

9. List five wearable medical devices.

_____

_____

_____

10. What serious challenges does the use of e-mail in healthcare present?

_____

_____

_____

11. Name five parts of the body that can be replaced by a prosthesis.

_____

_____

_____

12. How are lasers used to repair the body?

_____

_____

13. Which procedures can be performed using robotic surgery?

_____

_____

14. Why is cloning a controversial subject?

_____

_____

15. Which area of healthcare technology interests you the most? Why is this appealing to you?

_____

_____

_____

Fill in the Blanks: Healthcare Technology

Use the terms listed here to fill in the blanks in the following statements.

biotechnology	CT scan	genetic engineering	MRI
cloning	electronic health	handoff	prosthesis
computer	record (EHR)	HIPAA	robotic surgery
computer on wheels	electronic medical	HITECH	telemedicine
(COW)	record (EMR)		

1. A(n) _____ can serve a functional purpose, such as helping someone walk, or it can be purely cosmetic.

2. _____ is a controversial bioengineering development that creates an organism that is an exact genetic copy of another.

3. A(n) _____ uses a magnetic field and pulses of radio wave energy to make pictures of structures and organs inside the body.

4. Technology that uses biological processes, organisms, or systems to develop products intended to improve the quality of human life is called _____.

5. A patient's _____ contains information about his or her entire medical history and all of his or her healthcare experiences.

6. _____ reports are important during a shift change or a change in the level of patient care to explain a patient's current situation.

7. Modern healthcare technology is evident in _____, which involves the manipulation of genetic material to eliminate undesirable traits or ensure desirable traits.

8. During _____, the surgeon uses a computer to remotely control surgical instruments attached to a robot.

9. The _____ Act was passed in 2009 to improve healthcare through increased use of health information technology.

10. Due to the increase in technology, regardless of your position or occupation in healthcare, you will almost always use a(n) _____ to complete your tasks.

11. _____ is a field of medicine that uses telecommunication and information technologies to provide clinical health at a distance.

12. A(n) _____ allows healthcare workers to access and enter patient information while moving around a healthcare facility.

13. A medical imaging procedure called a(n) _____ allows organs to be seen in a cross direction.

14. A(n) _____ contains patient information from a single medical practice or even a single stay in one healthcare facility.

15. All healthcare workers must be familiar with _____ regulations that were passed by Congress in 1996 to protect the confidentiality of a patient's medical information.

Chapter 11

Vital Signs

Name _____ Date _____

What Is Normal?

Determine whether each of the following sets of vital signs is within the normal range for the specified individual. If they are normal, write normal *in the space provided. If they are not normal, explain which vital sign is not in the normal range and provide the normal range for that individual.*

1. Patrick is a 15-year-old male whose mother brought him to the clinic because he "just hasn't been feeling well."

    Vital signs: T—100.2°F (tympanic); P—82 bpm; R—16; BP—138/90

    Analysis: _____

2. Charlie is a 42-year-old male presenting with a runny nose, sore throat, and productive cough.

    Vital signs: T—102.4°F (oral); P—115 bpm; R—18; BP—128/82

    Analysis: _____

3. Jenna is an 18-month-old female brought to the clinic by her parents because she "just won't stop crying, so we know something must be wrong."

    Vital signs: T—100.8°F (rectal); P—110; R—46; BP—124/80

    Analysis: _____

4. Danyelle is a 61-year-old female who came into the doctor's office because she has been experiencing a "fluttering" feeling in her chest.

    Vital signs: T—36.6°C (oral); P—72; R—12; BP—102/64

    Analysis: _____

5. Bob is a 55-year-old hospital patient who had a complicated appendectomy yesterday.

    Vital signs: T—38.1°C (axillary); P—118; R—18; BP—140/94

    Analysis: _____

6. Harold is 3 weeks old and has a suspected ear infection.

    Vital signs: T—100.2°F (rectal); P—156; R—52; BP—80/58

    Analysis: _____

7. Lia is a 4-year-old whose mother brought her in for a checkup.

    Vital signs: T—99.4°F (temporal); P—132; R—32; BP—110/66

    Analysis: _____

8. Brad is a 17-year-old who was brought to the doctor's office because he fainted on the court yesterday during basketball practice.

    Vital signs: T—99.9°F (tympanic); P—46; R—26; BP—86/52

    Analysis: _____

Name _____   Date _____

Identifying Pulse Points

Label each pulse point on the image shown here.

1. _____

2. _____

3. _____

4. _____

5. _____

6. _____

7. _____

8. _____

9. _____

10. _____

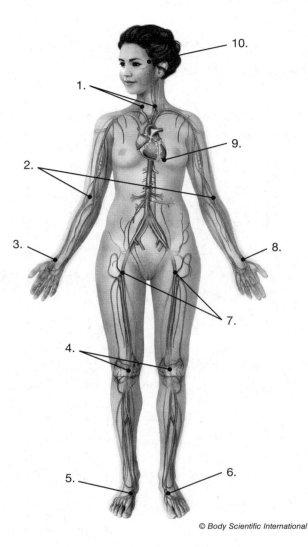

© Body Scientific International

Matching Vital Signs Terms

Match each of the following definitions with the correct term related to the vital signs. You will not use all of the terms.

_____ 1. body temperature below 95°F

_____ 2. temperature taken in the ear

_____ 3. difficult breathing observed as shortness of breath

_____ 4. a medical device used to measure blood pressure

_____ 5. excess retention or build-up of fluids in bodily tissues

_____ 6. an unusually slow rate of breathing

_____ 7. a long, thin medical instrument used to explore body cavities

_____ 8. temperature taken in the armpit

_____ 9. relating to the sense of hearing

_____ 10. breathing that sounds like snoring

_____ 11. a condition in which blood pressure is too high

_____ 12. lack of breathing

_____ 13. a pulse of less than 60 beats per minute

_____ 14. lack of adequate oxygen

_____ 15. rapid, shallow breathing due to the lungs only partially filling

A. apnea

B. aural

C. axillary temperature

D. bradycardia

E. bradypnea

F. dyspnea

G. edema

H. hypertension

I. hypothermia

J. hypoventilation

K. hypoxia

L. inhalation

M. probe

N. pulse oximeter

O. sphygmomanometer

P. stertorous breathing

Q. tachypnea

R. temporal artery temperature

S. tympanic temperature

It Takes More Than Technical Skill

Vital signs are called "vital" for a reason. They can give a healthcare worker vital, or critical, clues about a patient's condition. Unfortunately, the list of factors that can affect a person's vital signs is long, and it can be difficult to get a correct reading of those vital signs. No two patients are the same. Each individual has a different background, different beliefs, and even a different set of fears. Anger, fear, and excitement can affect the vital signs, so the patient should remain quiet and calm while you perform your assessment.

To get a good reading of a patient's vital signs, you will need to assess each patient individually. You may need to change your approach to keep the patient calm and still while you perform the assessment. Read each of the following scenarios and explain what you would do to obtain an accurate reading of each patient's vital signs.

1. Your patient is a 45-year-old male with a height of 5'8" and a weight of 332 lb. He seems uneasy while you are taking his tympanic temperature and recording his respirations. You have trouble finding the radial pulse because of the fatty deposits on his arms, but you are finally able to get a reading. When you try to wrap the regular blood pressure cuff around his arm, however, it doesn't reach all the way around. The patient is very embarrassed and starts stammering about how he knows he needs to lose weight. How will you handle this situation?

   _____

   _____

   _____

   _____

   _____

   _____

   _____

2. Your patient is a 3-year-old female who is grasping her left ear and crying loudly. She is obviously in pain, and when you ask if her ear hurts, she just cries harder. You need to get a complete set of vital signs, but you know that each vital sign will be affected by the child's distress. How will you handle this situation?

   _____

   _____

   _____

   _____

   _____

   _____

   _____

(Continued)

3. Your patient is a 15-year-old male brought in by his mother because of recent, unexplained weight loss. He tells his mother he doesn't want her to accompany him into the exam room, and she agrees to wait in the reception area. As you lead him to the exam room, it becomes apparent that he has an "attitude." He makes rude comments as you explain that you will check his vital signs. Nevertheless, he allows you to check his tympanic temperature, pulse, and respirations. For some reason, he goes wild when you approach him with the blood pressure cuff. He begins swearing and declaring that you are not going to put "that thing" on his arm. How will you handle this situation?

_____

_____

_____

_____

_____

_____

_____

4. Your patient is an 87-year-old female brought in by her daughter with a severe laceration on her left foot. The patient is shaking uncontrollably and seems to be afraid of her daughter. The daughter explains that her mother has dementia, which causes her to become paranoid. She says the laceration occurred when her mother was trying to help prepare dinner and dropped a sharp kitchen knife. The patient appears to understand when you explain what you are about to do, and she helps you roll up the sleeve of her shirt so that you can check her blood pressure. As she rolls up her sleeve, you notice bruises in various stages of healing. How will you handle this situation?

_____

_____

_____

_____

_____

_____

_____

_____

Understanding Hypotension

Partly due to dietary habits, hypertension is much more common today than hypotension. However, hypotension can also have major health consequences. Conduct research to find out more about the causes and symptoms of severe hypotension. Then answer the following questions. List your sources at the bottom of the page. Be sure to use reputable sources.

1. What are the possible causes of severe hypotension?

   _____

   _____

   _____

2. List and describe at least two different types of hypotension.

   _____

   _____

   _____

   _____

3. What are the symptoms of hypotension?

   _____

   _____

   _____

4. What tests are performed to determine the underlying cause of hypotension?

   _____

   _____

   _____

5. What treatments are available for hypotension?

   _____

   _____

   _____

Sources: _____

_____

_____

Documenting Vital Signs

Clear, concise, and complete documentation is an important element of assessing a patient's vital signs. Your documentation forms the basis for patient care, communicating essential information about the patient's health status to other healthcare workers involved in the patient's care. Many facilities have standard forms on which you can record your findings. In other cases, you may simply be expected to record the information in the patient's chart or EMR.

Remember that vital signs are not just a set of numbers. A patient's pulse, for example, may be regular or irregular, bounding or thready. These qualities need to be documented. Notice the depth and rhythm of a patient's respirations, as well as any abnormal sounds, such as wheezing. For temperature, you should always record the location used. Although some facilities assume an oral temperature if no location is given, it is always best to be specific, especially as tympanic thermometers have come into common use in medical offices. If you use a pulse oximeter, record the location where you placed the device. Always record any unusual circumstances that existed while you were assessing the patient.

Working with two other classmates, practice documenting vital signs. Assess each classmate's vital signs and document them correctly. Assume that your facility does not have a standard form for vital signs documentation. Include all relevant data about each vital sign.

Classmate #1

Temperature: _____

_____

Pulse: _____

_____

Respirations: _____

_____

Blood pressure: _____

_____

Classmate #2

Temperature: _____

_____

Pulse: _____

_____

Respirations: _____

_____

Blood pressure: _____

_____

Name _____   Date _____

Understanding First Aid and CPR

Answer the following questions.

1. What is first aid?

   _____

   _____

   _____

2. Provide five examples of emergency situations.

   _____

   _____

   _____

   _____

3. Why is timing so crucial in an emergency situation?

   _____

   _____

   _____

4. If you call 9-1-1 in an emergency situation, what guidelines should you follow when speaking to a 9-1-1 dispatcher?

   _____

   _____

   _____

   _____

   _____

5. Why is the use of protective gloves and a mask important when providing first aid?

   _____

   _____

   _____

(Continued)

6. As a general rule, you should not move someone who is injured. When should an injured person be moved?

_____

_____

7. What do the letters in the term *CPR* mean?

_____

8. Healthcare workers must be properly trained to perform CPR. Why is it a good idea to know CPR even if you are not working in a healthcare environment?

_____

_____

_____

9. What does the term *cardiac arrest* mean?

_____

_____

10. What does the term *respiratory arrest* mean?

_____

_____

11. When the situation calls for it, why is it important to start CPR as soon as possible?

_____

_____

_____

12. What does the term *hands-only CPR* mean?

_____

_____

13. What does the acronym *CAB* represent in reference to CPR?

_____

_____

14. Where and how should the hands be placed to perform chest compressions?

_____

_____

_____

(Continued)

15. When performing conventional CPR, how many chest compressions should you perform consecutively without interruptions?

_____

16. When performing rescue breathing, how should you open the airway?

_____

_____

_____

17. How many rescue breaths are given during CPR?

_____

18. In reference to a first aid emergency, what do the letters *AED* stand for?

_____

19. In what situation would you use an AED?

_____

_____

_____

20. List the steps for properly using an AED.

_____

_____

_____

_____

_____

_____

_____

_____

_____

_____

_____

Understanding Emergencies

Answer the following questions.

1. What is anaphylaxis?

   _____

   _____

   _____

2. List five common symptoms of anaphylaxis.

   _____

   _____

   _____

   _____

   _____

3. What should you do if someone experiences anaphylaxis?

   _____

   _____

   _____

   _____

   _____

   _____

4. List four ways poisons can enter the body.

   _____

   _____

   _____

   _____

   _____

(Continued)

5. List eight signs and symptoms of poisoning.

_____

_____

_____

_____

_____

_____

_____

_____

6. What is the number for the Poison Control Center?

_____

7. What are the signs and symptoms of an internal hemorrhage?

_____

_____

_____

_____

8. What is the universal sign for choking?

_____

_____

9. What is the Heimlich maneuver?

_____

_____

_____

_____

10. What is the rule of nines and how is it used?

_____

_____

_____

_____

_____

(Continued)

Name _____ Date _____

11. List the three degrees of burns in order from least severe to most severe.

_____

_____

_____

12. What is syncope and what causes it?

_____

_____

_____

_____

13. What is a seizure and what might cause one?

_____

_____

_____

_____

_____

14. What is the difference between a petit mal seizure and a grand mal seizure?

_____

_____

_____

_____

_____

_____

15. What is the primary consideration when trying to help someone who is experiencing a seizure?

_____

_____

_____

Name _____   Date _____

First Aid Terminology

Match each of the following definitions with the correct term related to first aid. You will not use all of the terms.

_____ 1. an event described as a sudden change in the brain's normal electrical activity that causes an altered or loss of consciousness

_____ 2. a medical device that delivers an electrical shock through the chest to the heart to stop an irregular heart rhythm and allow a normal heart rhythm to resume

_____ 3. an alternative procedure for those not trained in conventional CPR that uses uninterrupted chest compressions to restore the heartbeat and promote blood circulation

_____ 4. a drug that slows down or stops the actions of histamine, the substance that causes an allergic reaction

_____ 5. a method of calculating the surface area of the body that has been affected by a burn

_____ 6. a brief loss of consciousness that is considered a medical emergency; also known as *fainting* or *passing out*

_____ 7. a generalized seizure in which a person may experience a loss of consciousness and violent muscle contractions

_____ 8. a blue discoloration of the skin usually indicating a lack of oxygen and/or blood flow to the discolored tissue

_____ 9. a condition in which the body experiences a lack of sufficient oxygen available to the organs and tissues

_____ 10. a severe allergic reaction that can affect the whole body

_____ 11. excessive blood loss over a short period of time due to an internal or external injury

_____ 12. an irregular heart rhythm

_____ 13. a lack of oxygen that causes breathing to stop

_____ 14. a generalized seizure in which the person has impaired awareness and responsiveness, and may lose consciousness

_____ 15. a series of abdominal thrusts performed to remove an object that is lodged in a person's airway, preventing the person from breathing

A. allergen
B. anaphylaxis
C. antihistamine
D. asphyxia
E. automated external defibrillator (AED)
F. cardiopulmonary resuscitation (CPR)
G. cyanotic
H. fibrillation
I. grand mal seizure
J. hands-only CPR
K. Heimlich maneuver
L. hemorrhage
M. petit mal seizure
N. rule of nines
O. seizure
P. shock
Q. syncope

Knowing What to Do: CPR

Use your own words to describe the steps for properly performing CPR. As you do so, identify what each letter stands for in the acronym CAB.

C— _____

1. _____

_____

_____

_____

2. _____

_____

_____

_____

3. _____

_____

_____

_____

A— _____

4. _____

_____

_____

_____

_____

_____

_____

(Continued)

B— _____

5. _____

_____

_____

_____

_____

_____

_____

_____

6. _____

_____

_____

_____

_____

_____

_____

7. _____

_____

_____

_____

_____

_____

_____

Knowing What to Do: Anaphylaxis

Use your own words to describe the steps for handling an emergency situation that involves anaphylaxis.

1. _____
   _____
   _____
   _____
   _____

2. _____
   _____
   _____
   _____
   _____

3. _____
   _____
   _____
   _____
   _____

4. _____
   _____
   _____
   _____
   _____

5. _____
   _____
   _____
   _____
   _____

Knowing What to Do: Choking

Use your own words to describe the steps for handling an emergency situation that involves choking. Assume that the person involved in this emergency situation is a conscious adult.

1. _____
_____
_____

2. _____
_____
_____

3. _____
_____
_____

4. _____
_____
_____

5. _____
_____
_____

6. _____
_____
_____

7. _____
_____
_____

8. _____
_____
_____

9. _____
_____
_____

10. _____
_____

Knowing What to Do: Burns

Use your own words to describe what actions you should take in case of a third-degree burn. Assume that you have called 9-1-1 and are waiting for help to arrive.

1. _____
   _____
   _____
   _____
   _____
   _____
   _____

2. _____
   _____
   _____
   _____
   _____
   _____
   _____

3. _____
   _____
   _____
   _____
   _____
   _____
   _____

4. _____
   _____
   _____
   _____
   _____
   _____
   _____

5. _____
   _____
   _____
   _____
   _____
   _____

Name _____   Date _____

Knowing What to Do: Syncope

Use your own words to describe how you should respond to an emergency situation that involves syncope, or fainting.

1. _____
_____
_____

2. _____
_____
_____

3. _____
_____
_____

4. _____
_____
_____

5. _____
_____
_____

6. _____
_____
_____

7. _____
_____
_____

8. _____
_____
_____

9. _____
_____
_____

10. _____
_____
_____

Knowing What to Do: Seizures

Use your own words to describe the steps you should follow in an emergency situation that involves a severe seizure.

1. _____

_____

2. _____

_____

3. _____

_____

4. _____

_____

5. _____

_____

6. _____

_____

7. _____

_____

8. _____

_____

9. _____

_____

10. _____

_____

11. _____

_____

CPR Skills Worksheet

The following table can be used as a worksheet for assessing the skill requirements for performing CPR. Students should practice on a CPR skills trainer "manikin" only. Students should never simulate CPR on another student due to the potential of causing bodily harm.

If you have a certified CPR instructor on your campus, he or she will have access to CPR skills check-off sheets provided by an agency such as the American Heart Association or the American Red Cross. The table shown here is only a skills practice worksheet and is not endorsed by either of these organizations.

NAME: _____ **DATE:** _____

EVALUATOR: _____

SKILL	COMPLETED	NOT COMPLETED	TIME REQUIRED TO COMPLETE
Make sure it is safe to approach the victim.			
Check for responsiveness. (Tap the victim's shoulders and yell, "Are you OK?") (5–10 seconds)			
Have someone call 9-1-1. Have someone find the AED.			
Check for breathing and pulse (carotid). (5–10 seconds)			
Expose the chest before beginning compressions.			
CPR—use correct hand placement for compressions (lower half of the sternum)			
CPR—use correct depth for compressions (adult: 2–2 ½ inches)			
CPR—use correct rate for compressions (100–120 compressions per minute = 15–18 seconds)			
CPR—complete 30 compressions without stopping			
CPR—open the airway (head-tilt/chin-lift)			
CPR—provide 2 normal-sized breaths with good seal			
CPR—move back into position to start compressions (within 10 seconds)			
CPR—complete 5 sets of 30 compressions and 2 breaths			
Demonstrate the proper use of an AED.			

COMMENTS:

_____

_____

_____

_____

_____

Chapter 13

Assisting with Mobility

Name _____   Date _____

Identifying Range-of-Motion Exercises

Read the following scenarios and identify the body part that each therapist or patient is targeting with the exercises that are described. Then list the range-of-motion exercises that are typically performed on that body part.

1. The therapist asks Jim to lie on his side with his arms and hands positioned comfortably in front of him. The therapist uses her hand and arm to support Jim's upper knee, gently lifting his entire leg about 10 inches, and then slowly lowers it. She performs this exercise 10 times.

   Targeted body part: _____

   Typical range-of-motion exercises for this body part: _____

2. The therapist tells Eva to sit up straight in the chair with her hands at her sides. Grasping Eva's left arm at the elbow and the wrist, the therapist proceeds to lift the arm straight over Eva's head and then lowers it back down to her side. After five repetitions, he moves the arm straight out to the side, away from Eva's body, and then lowers it again to Eva's side. He does this for five repetitions as well.

   Targeted body part: _____

   Typical range-of-motion exercises for this body part: _____

3. The therapist holds Vance's wrist with both hands and gently bends his hand down, then up, then down again, for eight repetitions. Then she holds Vance's wrist in one hand and grasps his palm with her other hand. She turns the palm about 20° in the direction of the thumb, turns it back to its usual alignment with the arm, and then turns it the other way, toward the little finger. She does this for eight repetitions as well.

   Targeted body part: _____

   Typical range-of-motion exercises for this body part: _____

4. As directed by her physician, Tania holds her right foot at the ankle. With her other hand, she grasps the foot at a point that is medial to the toes and pulls upward while pushing down on the heel. She then reverses the actions, pulling up on the heel while pushing down on the foot. She does this for five repetitions.

   Targeted body part: _____

   Typical range-of-motion exercises for this body part: _____

5. While Janice is lying supine on the treatment table, the therapist places one hand under her left knee and supports her left ankle with his other hand. Slowly and smoothly, he moves the knee up and the ankle toward Janice's hip so that the knee bends. Then he slowly moves the leg back to its original position. He does this 10 times with Janice's left leg, and then repeats the process with Janice's right leg.

   Targeted body part: _____

   Typical range-of-motion exercises for this body part: _____

Scrambled Mobility Terms

Unscramble the letters in each item below to form a term related to mobility. Then define each term.

1. D R A I N C O N I T T E D C A

    Term: _____

    Definition: _____

2. B I D T U C U S E L U R E C

    Term: _____

    Definition: _____

3. T R O C C I E N

    Term: _____

    Definition: _____

4. N O L A S S I K Y

    Term: _____

    Definition: _____

5. C R A T H E N R O T L O L R

    Term: _____

    Definition: _____

6. N O R T T A C R U C E

    Term: _____

    Definition: _____

7. S L O B U M E

    Term: _____

    Definition: _____

8. B I M I O T Y L I M

    Term: _____

    Definition: _____

9. Y A N O T

    Term: _____

    Definition: _____

10. O R T T A C N I

    Term: _____

    Definition: _____

Practicing Safe Patient Handling

Read each of the following descriptions and identify what should have been done differently to ensure the safety of the healthcare worker and/or the patient.

1. After repositioning a patient, the healthcare worker routes the urinary catheter against the skin of the patient's left leg.

   _____

   _____

2. A CNA working in a hospital is asked to assist a woman who weighs 285 lb, has limited mobility, and needs help washing her back. The CNA uses a turning sheet to position the patient on her side.

   _____

   _____

3. While transferring a patient from a bed to a wheelchair, the technician stands with his feet together and grasps the patient's hands to help her stand from her current position sitting on the bed.

   _____

   _____

4. An unconscious patient is repositioned every four hours, as needed.

   _____

   _____

5. While repositioning a patient, the patient care technician crosses the patient's legs so that her injured foot is elevated on top of her other foot.

   _____

   _____

6. Before transferring an immobile patient to a stretcher, the healthcare workers adjust the bed to its lowest position.

   _____

   _____

7. The medical assistant twisted to the right and then to the left to help straighten the sheets around an immobilized patient's legs and shoulders.

   _____

   _____

8. While transferring a frail patient who has recently undergone abdominal surgery, the two healthcare workers grasp her arms and legs to avoid causing pain in the abdominal area.

   _____

   _____

Interpreting Abbreviations

Identify the meaning of each abbreviation or acronym in the following sentences. You may need to look up some of the abbreviations used.

1. One week after surgery, the surgeon's office called Mr. Jacobs to ask whether he had resumed his ADL.

   _____

2. The physician directed the patient to receive AAROM exercises q6h while awake.

   _____

   _____

3. The patient in room 3141 is to be OOB as much as possible and up ad lib.

   _____

   _____

4. Ms. Brookes is currently on BR with BRP.

   _____

   _____

5. After outpatient foot surgery, W/C transportation is ordered to move Mrs. White to her daughter's car. Her postoperative instructions state, "Amb as tolerated after two days."

   _____

   _____

6. For a patient with severe hypotension, the physician's order reads, "Elevate HOB 20°; Pt requires assistance when getting OOB."

   _____

   _____

7. One day after surgery, a patient who has had a TKA is placed on a CPM machine to exercise the leg.

   _____

   _____

8. A patient requires passive ROM for an injured hip. The physician's orders specify FADIR 3x daily.

   _____

   _____

Name _____ Date _____

Identifying Pressure Points

Carefully study each image shown here. Then label the potential pressure points, where decubitus ulcers are likely to develop, on each patient. Draw lines leading to each pressure point you identify and label each one with the body part affected.

1.

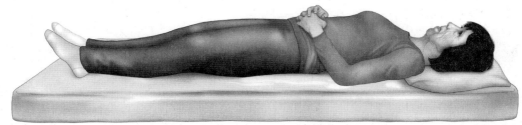

© Body Scientific International

2.

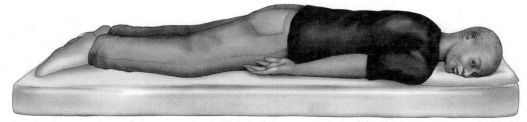

© Body Scientific International

3.

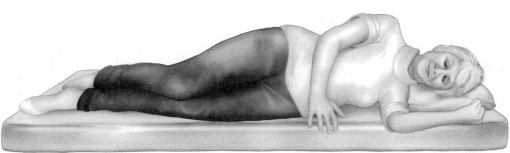

© Body Scientific International

4.

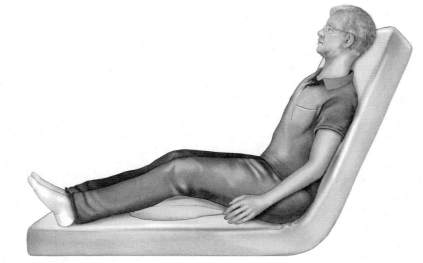

© Body Scientific International

Teaching Patients to Use Assistive Devices

Read each item below and answer the questions.

1. Study the gaits presented in the textbook for ambulating using a cane, crutches, and a walker. Choose one of these assistive devices and create a teaching plan to help a patient learn to use the device properly. Record your plan here.

   _____

   _____

   _____

   _____

   _____

2. Test your teaching plan on another student. Have the student simulate an injury or disability that requires the assistive device you chose, and then follow your instructions. How well did your plan work? Ask the student for constructive criticism. What could you have explained better? What else would have improved your presentation? Record ideas for refining your teaching plan here.

   _____

   _____

   _____

   _____

   _____

3. Revise your plan as necessary and test it on another student. Again, ask for feedback. Then conduct a discussion with both students about the potential issues that may occur when healthcare workers are teaching patients how to use assistive devices. Write a summary paragraph describing your conclusions.

   _____

   _____

   _____

   _____

   _____

   _____

Chapter 14

Working in Healthcare

Name _____ Date _____

Healthcare Terms Matching

Match each of the following definitions with the correct term.

_____ 1. term for actions taken to maintain oral health and prevent the spread of disease

_____ 2. the surgical opening or puncture of a vein to withdraw blood

_____ 3. the act of using the hands to feel an object, such as a lump on the body or a mass in the body, to determine its location, size, shape, and hardness

_____ 4. the term commonly used to indicate when a patient is released from or leaves the healthcare facility to go home

_____ 5. a medical device designed to enter a body opening such as the vagina, rectum, or nose, making those areas visible for an examination

_____ 6. a written or computer entry order for a medication to be prepared or filled in a pharmacy

_____ 7. a device used to examine the mouth, tongue, and teeth

_____ 8. a set of instructions regarding the patient's treatment and medications for use after leaving a healthcare facility

_____ 9. to assign the accountability and responsibility of one's task to another worker

_____ 10. a lighted medical device used to examine the interior of the eyes

_____ 11. the term commonly used to indicate when a patient is moved to a new location within the same healthcare facility or to a completely different facility

_____ 12. the act of using a stethoscope to listen to the internal sounds of the body, such as the heartbeat

_____ 13. a sticky substance found on teeth

_____ 14. a lighted medical device used to examine the ear and eardrum

_____ 15. the act of tapping on areas of the body to determine underlying body structure issues such as fluid in the abdominal or chest cavities

A. auscultation

B. delegate

C. discharge

D. discharge plan

E. laryngeal mirror

F. ophthalmoscope

G. oral prophylaxis

H. otoscope

I. palpation

J. percussion

K. phlebotomy

L. plaque

M. prescription

N. speculum

O. transfer

Positioning and Draping For Physical Examinations

When planning or preparing for a physical examination, medical personnel must be familiar with specific positions in which to place the patient, as well as proper draping techniques to allow access to the area being examined, maintain patient dignity, and make the patient feel as comfortable as possible. Each practitioner and each facility might have specific protocols for patient positions during physical examinations. It is the job of the healthcare worker to learn individual protocols. Read each of the descriptions in the table below and identify the correct patient position.

Description of Positioning and Draping	Position
In this position, the patient lies on his or her left side, with the lower arm bent behind the back. The upper knee is bent and raised toward the chest and supported by a pillow. A pillow is also placed under the foot so the toes do not touch the table. The drape extends from the shoulder to the toes. This position is used to examine the rectum or vagina.	
In this position, the patient is seated on the table with the table at a 45-degree angle. The legs are extended flat on the table. The drape should cover the legs, if necessary. This position is often used to examine the legs and feet.	
This position has the patient lie on the abdomen (stomach) with the arms and hands to each side and the head turned to the side. The drape extends from the shoulders to the legs and may cover the feet. This position is used to examine the spine and legs.	
In this position, the patient kneels on the table with the head and chest remaining on the table and the buttocks raised. The arms are extended above the head with the elbows bent. The head is turned to one side and a pillow can be placed under the chest. The drape covers the back and legs. This position is used to examine the rectum.	
This position has the patient lie on the back with the arms at each side. The drape extends from under the armpits to the toes. This position is used for examination of the front of the body and breasts.	
In this position, the patient is flat on the back with the knees bent and feet flat on the table. The drape is placed in a diamond shape, covering the chest and extending down to cover the perineal area (between the anus and the scrotum on the male, and between the anus and the opening to the vagina on the female). This position is used to examine the rectum and vagina.	
This position is typically used for female patients. The patient lies on her back, with her hips brought to the end (corners) of the table. Her legs are bent and her feet are placed in padded stirrups. The drape is placed in a diamond shape, covering the body from the chest down to the perineal area. This position is typically used to examine the vagina.	

Examination Equipment

Match each of the following descriptions with the correct piece of equipment. You will not use all of the terms.

_____ 1. a device used to determine a patient's body temperature

_____ 2. a lighted medical device used to examine the interior of the eyes

_____ 3. a device used to test hearing

_____ 4. common protective equipment used to prevent the hands from coming in contact with infectious body fluids

_____ 5. a device used to measure a patient's blood pressure; also known as a *blood pressure cuff*

_____ 6. a medical device designed to enter a body opening such as the vagina, rectum, or nose, making those areas visible for an examination

_____ 7. a device used to examine the mouth, tongue, and teeth

_____ 8. a simple, disposable medical device, usually a thin strip of wood, used to press the tongue down to examine the throat

_____ 9. a common device used to shine light into the eyes to evaluate the pupils for dilation

_____ 10. a medical device used to tap body parts to test reflexes

_____ 11. a lighted medical device used to examine the ear and eardrum

_____ 12. a medical device used to measure blood pressure, heart and lung sounds, and pulse

A. disposable gloves
B. eye chart
C. flashlight
D. laryngeal mirror
E. ophthalmoscope
F. otoscope
G. percussion (reflex) hammer
H. speculum
I. sphygmomanometer
J. stethoscope
K. thermometer
L. tongue depressor
M. tuning fork

Understanding Healthcare Careers

Identify the roles, responsibilities, and education and training requirements for each of the following healthcare careers, which are explored in chapter 14.

1. nursing assistant

   Roles and Responsibilities: _____

   _____

   _____

   Education and Training Requirements: _____

   _____

   _____

2. patient care technician

   Roles and Responsibilities: _____

   _____

   _____

   Education and Training Requirements: _____

   _____

   _____

3. health unit coordinator (HUC)

   Roles and Responsibilities: _____

   _____

   _____

   Education and Training Requirements: _____

   _____

   _____

4. medical assistant

   Roles and Responsibilities: _____

   _____

   _____

   Education and Training Requirements: _____

   _____

   _____

(Continued)

5. dental assistant

   Roles and Responsibilities: _____

   _____

   _____

   Education and Training Requirements: _____

   _____

   _____

6. pharmacy technician

   Roles and Responsibilities: _____

   _____

   _____

   Education and Training Requirements: _____

   _____

   _____

7. physical therapy assistant

   Roles and Responsibilities: _____

   _____

   _____

   Education and Training Requirements: _____

   _____

   _____

8. emergency medical technician (EMT)

   Roles and Responsibilities: _____

   _____

   _____

   Education and Training Requirements: _____

   _____

   _____

Name _____ Date _____

Admission Procedure

Using the information found in Procedure 14.1 on pages 420–421 of your textbook, provide a brief description of the full admission procedure. You may combine several steps as they are listed in the text, but be sure to include something for each of the four categories—preparation, procedure, follow-up, and reporting and documentation.

Preparation

_____

_____

_____

_____

_____

_____

_____

_____

Procedure

_____

_____

_____

_____

_____

_____

_____

_____

_____

Follow-Up

_____

_____

_____

Reporting and Documentation

_____

_____

_____

Transfer Procedure

Using the information found in Procedure 14.2 on page 422 of your textbook, provide a brief description of the full transfer procedure. You may combine several steps as they are listed in the text, but be sure to include something for each of the four categories—preparation, procedure, follow-up, and reporting and documentation.

Preparation

_____

_____

_____

_____

_____

_____

_____

Procedure

_____

_____

_____

_____

_____

_____

_____

_____

_____

Follow-Up

_____

_____

_____

Reporting and Documentation

_____

_____

_____

Discharge Procedure

Using the information found in Procedure 14.3 on pages 423–424, provide a brief description of the full discharge procedure. You may combine several steps as they are listed in the text, but be sure to include something for each of the four categories—preparation, procedure, follow-up, and reporting and documentation.

Preparation

_____

_____

_____

_____

_____

_____

_____

_____

_____

Procedure

_____

_____

_____

_____

_____

_____

_____

_____

_____

Follow-Up

_____

_____

_____

Reporting and Documentation

_____

_____

_____

Chapter 15

Communication Skills

Name _____ Date _____

Taking Telephone Messages

Read the following transcripts of telephone conversations that include Fran, who is a receptionist at a busy clinic, and various patients. Then, for each conversation, write an appropriate message directed to the appropriate person. Be sure to include all of the necessary information. If no message is required, write, No message required.

1. Call log: Tuesday, 2/16/2017, 9:42 a.m.

Fran: "Good morning, Marlow Clinic, this is Fran. How may I help you?"

Caller: "Hello, this is Brenda Young, and I think my daughter may have an ear infection. What should I do?"

Fran: "Ms. Young, how old is your daughter?"

Caller: "She is two and a half years old, and she just won't stop crying."

Fran: "The best thing would be to bring her in to see one of the doctors. Can you bring her into the office this afternoon at 3:00 p.m.?"

Caller: "No, we are out of town on vacation. I can call you back for an appointment on Thursday. What can I do for her in the meantime? Can you have Dr. Snyder call me?"

Fran: "What is your daughter's name and birthday? Has she been seen in this clinic before?"

Caller: "Her name is Sonja Young, and her birthday is August 16, 2014. She has been there before. Dr. Snyder is her regular pediatrician."

Fran: "Okay, is that 'S-O-N-Y-A Y-O-U-N-G'?"

Caller: "No, it's S-O-N-J-A."

Fran: "And at what number can we reach you?"

Caller: "Please call my cell phone at 555-122-4867."

Fran: "That was 555-122-4867, correct? I will leave a message for Dr. Snyder, but in the meantime, you may want to consider taking Sonja to the closest urgent care center for treatment."

_____

_____

_____

_____

2. Call log: Tuesday, 2/16/2017, 11:55 a.m.

Fran: "Good morning, Marlow Clinic, this is Fran. How may I help you?"

Caller: "My name is Donna Winters. I was told to call today to find out the results of the tests Dr. Craig ordered on Monday."

Fran: "Hello, Ms. Winters. May I have your date of birth?"

Caller: "My birthday is 9/25/1993."

(Continued)

Fran: "Thank you. May I put you on hold for a moment while I check with Dr. Craig?"

Caller: "Yes, thank you."

[Fran puts the caller on hold…]

Fran: "Ms. Winters?"

Caller: "Yes?"

Fran: "I am happy to report that Dr. Craig has received all of your test results, and they are all normal."

Caller: "Oh, that is good news! Thank you very much!"

_____

_____

3. **Call log: Tuesday, 2/16/2017, 1:15 p.m.**

   Fran: "Good afternoon, Marlow Clinic, this is Fran. How may I help you?"

   Caller: "Good afternoon, Fran, this is Dr. Robert Wilson at Tricorner Medical Center. Is Dr. Trent available?"

   Fran: "Hi, Dr. Wilson. Dr. Trent is with a patient right now. May I have him call you back?"

   Caller: "Yes, please. Ask him to call me at 555-523-8142 about Shelley Underwood, DOB 11/5/1962, a referral he sent me last week."

   Fran: "Okay, that's 555-523-8142, and the patient's name is 'S-H-E-L-L-E-Y U-N-D-E-R-W-O-O-D,' correct?"

   Caller: "Yes, thank you. I would like to discuss this case with him as soon as possible."

   Fran: "I will give him the message. Thank you for calling."

   _____

   _____

   _____

   _____

4. **Call log: Tuesday, 2/16/2017, 2:34 p.m.**

   Fran: "Good afternoon, Marlow Clinic, this is Fran. How may I help you?"

   Caller: "My name is David Murdock. Dr. Trent told me to call today to let him know how the antibiotic worked. I am happy to report that I feel much better."

   Fran: "That is wonderful to hear, Mr. Murdock. Can you please confirm your date of birth?"

   Caller: "I'm not sure why you need to know, but my birthday is May 3, 1955."

   Fran: "We use your date of birth to avoid any confusion with other patients who have similar names, and to make sure that we record the information in the correct chart. I will give Dr. Trent the message, and I am glad you are feeling better. Please let us know if your condition worsens or if you have any questions."

   _____

   _____

   _____

   _____

Understanding Communication

Use the terms listed here to fill in the blanks in the following statements. You will not use all of the terms.

active	concise	objective	sarcasm	verbal
aphasia	etiquette	open-ended	sender-receiver	
barriers	noise	passive	stereotype	
closed	nonverbal	proxemics	subjective	

1. The study of _____ can help you understand a person's sense of physical territory and personal territory.

2. Telephone _____ includes how you speak and behave while talking on the telephone.

3. Communication between two people can be described using the _____ communication model.

4. Anything that interferes with a person's understanding of a message, creating a barrier to communication, can be described as _____.

5. Body language is another term for _____ communication.

6. _____ writing emphasizes a person's feelings or opinions.

7. Imagine you are trying to talk to a patient, but a child is crying loudly nearby and the telephone is ringing. These environmental factors are considered _____ to communication.

8. Technical writing is considered a type of _____ writing because it is based on evidence that can be seen and evaluated.

9. A person who listens in an attempt not just to hear your words but also to understand the complete message you are sending is engaging in _____ listening.

10. A stroke is a common cause of a collection of language disorders known as _____, which are caused by brain damage.

11. It is important to avoid using _____ when you are working with patients because they may misunderstand or take your meaning literally.

12. Asking _____ questions instead of questions that require only a *yes* or *no* response is a good way to gain more information from a patient.

13. The process of expressing thoughts by speaking them aloud is known as _____ communication.

14. An assumption or judgment about a group of people or a situation that is based on a limited amount of information is called a(n) _____ and should be avoided when working with patients and other healthcare workers.

15. The *5 Cs of Communication* are clear, credible, _____, courteous, and consistent.

Name _____ Date _____

Professional E-mail Communication

Read the e-mail messages shown here, each of which was written by an office staff member at the request of a licensed practitioner. Assume that each healthcare facility has signed permission on file allowing e-mail communications with each of these patients. Circle any errors or problems you find in each message, and then use the space provided to offer suggestions for improvement.

1.

> **To:** Denise Remington
> **Subject:** Your Pap smear results
>
> Hi, Denise! My name is Rene Wilson, and I am a medical assistant at Dr. Jenkins' office. Dr. Jenkins wanted me to let you know that the Pap smear was normal, but it looks like you have a slight yeast infection. She wants you to use an over-the-counter three-day coarse of Monistat to help clear it up. Please let us know if u have any questions.
>
> Sincerely,
> Rene Wilson, CMA
> Upstate OB/GYN, LLC

_____

_____

_____

2.

> **To:** Geri Markham, MD
> **Subject:** Question
>
> Dr. Markham:
>
> Dr. Haskell wanted me to confirm that you will be able to address the local chapter of the AMA on Thursday evening. We know your schedule is busy, but Dr. Haskell believes you have much to contribute to this meeting, which focuses on resent changes in orthopedic surgerical techniques. Please let us know as soon as possible whether you will be joining us.
>
> Thank you,
> Cindy Thompson, RMA
> Orthopedic Associates, Ltd.

_____

_____

_____

(Continued)

3.

> **To**: Daniel W. Putnam
>
> **Subject**: Time for Your Annual Exam!
>
> Dear Mr. Putnam:
>
> It is hard to believe an entire year has passed! But time flies, and it is time to schedule your annual wellness exam. We at New Verizons Clinic believe that every patient requires a wellness exam at least annually, and we strongly urge you to make an appointment today. You never know what might happen in a year's time! If you have any lurking problems, the sooner we find them, the sooner we can fix them. In addition, when we find health problems in their early stages, they are much easier to treat.
>
> Although your last physical exam showed that you were in perfect health, due to your advanced age, our physicians will do a thorough exam, including bloodwork, a urinalysis, an electrocardiogram, and a rectal exam. We realize that cardiac problems and colon cancer run in your family. Statistics show that men over the age of 50 who have a family history of either of these conditions are at a greater risk of developing them, and we want to take the best possible care of you.
>
> Please contact our office today at 555-828-6691 to set up an appointment with any one of our experienced physicians.

_____

_____

_____

_____

Objective Writing

Read each of the following patient encounters. Then practice writing objectively by creating an objective assessment as directed. You may use appropriate abbreviations.

1. On January 28, 2017, Penny Hightower comes to the physician's office because she is having abdominal pain. She says she has been having the pain for three days now, and that it is concentrated just below her navel on the right side. She says, "It feels like someone is sticking a knife in me! Sometimes I can barely move!" When asked to rate her pain on a scale of 1 to 10, she rates it as an 8. She states that she thinks she has appendicitis. Write a note for Penny's chart describing this information.

   Chart note: _____

   _____

   _____

   _____

   _____

   _____

   _____

   _____

2. At 3:40 p.m. on June 16, 2017, Darryl Strombourg is brought to the urgent care clinic with a bleeding laceration on his left arm. Even though the medical assistant, Sherri Blakely, quickly puts on gloves and attempts to stop the flow of blood, quite a bit of blood drips onto the floor. As Sherri escorts the patient to an exam room, he slips in the blood and falls, injuring his left knee. He cannot stand up, even with Sherri's help, and he says he thinks his knee is dislocated. The patient is furious, saying he came in for medical help and now he has twice as many problems as when he arrived. Sherri calls on her coworkers Willi Brandon, RNA, and David Lofton, EMT-P, to help. Together they place Darryl on a stretcher and take him to an exam room, where the physician on duty sees him immediately. Write an incident report about this accident to present to your supervisor.

   Incident report: _____

   _____

   _____

   _____

   _____

   _____

   _____

   _____

   _____

Oral Presentation

Choose a common but preventable disease or healthcare issue that interests you. Conduct research to find out more about the topic. Be sure to use reputable sources. Record your notes below. Then prepare a three-minute oral presentation to persuade listeners to take the necessary steps to prevent the disease or healthcare issue. With a partner, take turns practicing your oral presentations. Provide each other with constructive criticism to improve the persuasiveness of your presentations. Be prepared to present your persuasive speech in class.

Disease or healthcare issue: _____

Research notes: _____

_____

_____

_____

_____

Presentation notes: _____

_____

_____

_____

_____

_____

Critique: _____

_____

_____

_____

_____

_____

Sources: _____

_____

_____

_____

Nonverbal Communication

Although you may rarely need to use it, knowing American Sign Language (ASL) can help you communicate more effectively with hearing-impaired patients. The ASL alphabet is reproduced below. Study the alphabet and become familiar with the various hand positions. Then create a one-sentence message of at least 10 words to be expressed using only ASL. After you practice delivering your message in front of a mirror, test your skill by delivering your message to a partner. Then have your partner deliver a message to you.

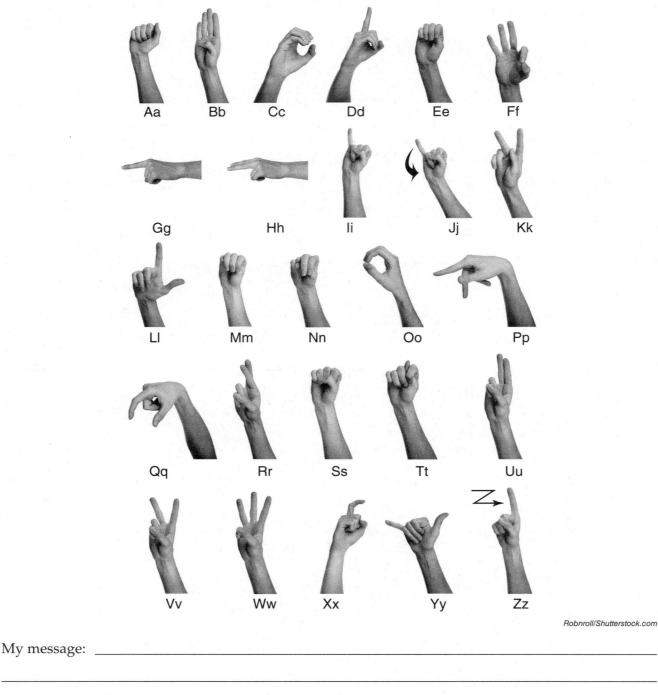

Robnroll/Shutterstock.com

My message: _____

_____

My partner's message: _____

Chapter 16

Medical Math Skills

Name _____ Date _____

Math Terms Matching

Match each of the following definitions with the correct term.

_____ 1. the unit of measurement that indicates a drug's weight or action

_____ 2. a mathematical expression that compares one quantity with another, similar quantity

_____ 3. the number exactly in the middle of a group of numbers listed in ascending or descending order

_____ 4. the branch of mathematics that substitutes letters for numbers to solve for unknown quantities

_____ 5. an amount per one hundred

_____ 6. the official name assigned to a drug in the United States

_____ 7. a method of measuring time based on 24-hour long segments; also called *military time*

_____ 8. a statement of the equality of two ratios

_____ 9. fractions that are expressed in the base 10 system; also known as *decimal fractions*

_____ 10. letters used by the ancient Romans to represent numbers

_____ 11. the mathematical average of data

_____ 12. the name assigned to a drug by its manufacturer

_____ 13. the dosage strength of a drug; describes the amount of medication per administration unit

_____ 14. the number that occurs most frequently in a set of numbers

_____ 15. a method of measuring time based on a 12-hour system in which a.m. and p.m. designations must be assigned to identify the proper time

A. 12-hour clock
B. 24-hour clock
C. algebra
D. concentration
E. decimals
F. dosage unit
G. generic name
H. mean
I. median
J. mode
K. percentage
L. proportion
M. ratio
N. Roman numerals
O. trade name

Understanding Math Terms

Use the terms listed here to fill in the blanks in the following statements.

12-hour clock	database	expiration date	percentage
24-hour clock	English system of measurement	metric system of measurement	spreadsheet
administration units	equation	on-hand dose	trade name

1. A(n) _____ is a document containing rows and columns of data that is useful for organizing numeric values and performing computer calculations.

2. Two sides of a(n) _____ are separated by an equal sign and must be equal to one another.

3. A(n) _____ for a medication varies from one company to another and is assigned to a drug by its manufacturer.

4. Tablets, capsules, teaspoons, tablespoons, ounces, drops, liters, and milliliters are considered the most common _____.

5. The _____ requires the use of a.m. and p.m. designations to identify the proper time.

6. The _____ uses units related by factors of 10, including grams, liters, meters, and Celsius degrees.

7. When documenting meal intake, a nursing assistant might use a(n) _____ to document how much of the meal the patient ate.

8. A(n) _____ is a detailed collection of related information, organized for convenient access, generally by a digital device.

9. In the healthcare world, time is often expressed using the _____, which is commonly known as *military time.*

10. The date placed on a container of medication that indicates when the medication is no longer fit for use is known as the _____.

11. The _____ is commonly used in the United States and is based on units such as the inch, pound, gallon, and Fahrenheit degrees.

12. The amount of medication per capsule or other delivery method is referred to as the _____.

Name _____ Date _____

Fractions, Decimals, and Ratios

Provide the missing fraction, written description, or decimal to complete each row in the table shown here.

Fraction	Written Description	Decimal
1/10		
	one-hundredth	
		.001
	one ten-thousandth	
1/1,000,000		
	one-fifth	
		.5

Convert the following fractions to decimals. Round to the nearest hundredth, if necessary. You may complete these on a separate sheet of paper so you can show your work without using a calculator.

1. 2/3 =

2. 5/8 =

3. 1/4 =

4. 5/6 =

5. 8/9 =

6. 3/7 =

7. 3/6 =

8. 2/9 =

9. 2/5 =

10. 1/5 =

(Continued)

Name _____ Date _____

Convert the following fractions into decimals and percentages without the use of a calculator.

11. 3/13

    Decimal: _____

    Percentage: _____

12. 4/15

    Decimal: _____

    Percentage: _____

13. 7/10

    Decimal: _____

    Percentage: _____

14. 1/4

    Decimal: _____

    Percentage: _____

15. 1 1/4

    Decimal: _____

    Percentage: _____

16. 3/5

    Decimal: _____

    Percentage: _____

Identify the simplest form of each of the following ratios.

17. 20:15: _____

18. 10:5: _____

19. 4:6: _____

20. 8:32: _____

Algebra and Medications

Solve for the unknown quantity indicated by the x in each of the following algebraic equations. Show your work.

1. $x + 6 = 10$

2. $2x - 10 = 10$

3. $5x - 5 = 10$

4. $4x = 60$

5. $5x = 100$

6. $3x + 8 = 20$

7. $50 - 3x = 20$

8. $10 + 25 - 15 = 5x$

9. $6x + 9 - 10 = 5$

10. $200 - 46 + 50 - 60 = 12x$

(Continued)

Name _____   Date _____

Use the formula D/H x Q = amount to be administered *to solve each of the following word problems.*

> ORDER: A vial of medicine has 200 mg of medicine in each 1 mL. The doctor has ordered the patient to receive 400 mg of the medicine to be given 4 times a day.

11. How many milliliters of the medicine should be given at each dose? _____

12. What is the total amount of medicine to be given in a day? _____

> ORDER: The doctor has ordered for a patient to receive 1,000 units of a medication. The medication bottle states that there are 200 units per 1 mL of the medication.

13. How many milliliters of the medication should be given to the patient?

   _____

14. If the bottle of medication contains a total volume of 50 mL, how many doses could be given

   from this bottle, assuming that each dose is an equal amount? _____

> ORDER: The doctor has issued an order for 25 mg of a medication to be given in a dose 4 times a day. The medication comes in a scored tablet with each tablet containing 10 mg of the medication.

15. How many tablets are given in each dose? _____

16. How many tablets should be given per day? _____

17. If you have a supply of 50 tablets available, how long will the supply last at the current dose rate?

   _____

Write an algebraic equation for the following problem, and then use your equation to solve the problem.

18. The doctor orders you to give a double dose of a medication and a 10 mL dose of a second medication to a patient. The total amount of medicine to be administered to the patient is 50 mL. What is the standard, single dose of the first medication?

Name _____ Date _____

Using Mean, Median, and Mode

Answer the following questions.

1. Determine the mean, median, and mode of the following series of numbers.

   24   36   48   48   52   66   72   84

   mean = _____

   median = _____

   mode = _____

2. A patient was admitted to the hospital due to hypertension. The following blood pressure readings were recorded for the patient over a 24-hour period.

   150/94   160/110   154/100   142/90   154/100   166/120

   Determine the mean, median, and mode for the systolic and diastolic blood pressure readings.

   systolic mean = _____

   systolic median = _____

   systolic mode = _____

   diastolic mean = _____

   diastolic median = _____

   diastolic mode = _____

3. Northtown Hospital is evaluating its patient admissions over the past six months. Identify the mean, median, and mode of the following admission totals.

   Jan = 498   Feb = 480   Mar = 488   Apr = 480   May = 464   Jun = 470

   mean = _____

   median = _____

   mode = _____

Metric and English Unit Conversions

Provide the multiples of one for the following metric prefixes.

EXAMPLE: giga- = 1,000,000,000

1. kilo- = _____   3. mega- = _____

2. deca- = _____   4. hecto- = _____

Provide the multiples of one (fraction) and the decimal equivalency for the following metric prefixes.

EXAMPLE: nano- = 1/1,000,000,000 = .000000001

5. deci- = _____ = _____

6. micro- = _____ = _____

7. milli- = _____ = _____

8. centi- = _____ = _____

Convert the following units within the metric system.

9. 1 gram = _____ milligrams   12. 1 gram = _____ centigrams

10. 1 gram = _____ kilograms   13. 1 meter = _____ centimeters

11. 1 gram = _____ micrograms   14. 1 liter = _____ milliliters

Convert the following units within the English system.

15. 1 pound = _____ ounces   18. 1 mile = _____ feet

16. 1 foot = _____ inches   19. 1 quart = _____ pints

17. 1 yard = _____ feet   20. 1 tablespoon = _____ teaspoons

Convert the following English units to metric units.

21. 10 inches = _____ centimeters

22. 100 feet = _____ meters

23. 10 ounces = _____ grams

24. 100 ounces = _____ kilograms

25. 100 pounds = _____ kilograms

26. 10 teaspoons = _____ milliliters

27. 10 fluid ounces = _____ milliliters

28. 100 cups = _____ liters

29. 10 pints = _____ liters

30. 10 gallons = _____ liters

Converting Temperature and Time

Convert the following temperatures from Fahrenheit to Celsius.

1. 98.6 = _____

2. 100 = _____

3. 106 = _____

4. 97 = _____

5. 32 = _____

6. 212 = _____

Convert the following temperatures from Celsius to Fahrenheit.

7. 98.6 = _____

8. 50 = _____

9. 112 = _____

10. 75 = _____

11. 0 = _____

12. 100 = _____

Convert the following times from the 12-hour clock to the 24-hour clock.

13. 8:05 a.m. = _____

14. 8:05 p.m. = _____

15. 12:30 a.m. = _____

16. 12:30 p.m. = _____

17. 4:00 a.m. = _____

18. 4:00 p.m. = _____

19. 10:45 a.m. = _____

20. 10:45 p.m. = _____

Convert the following times from the 24-hour clock to the 12-hour clock.

21. 2355 = _____

22. 1620 = _____

23. 0800 = _____

24. 1111 = _____

25. 0910 = _____

26. 1245 = _____

27. 1730 = _____

28. 2110 = _____

29. 0130 = _____

30. 0545 = _____

Chapter 17

Study Skills

Name _____ Date _____

Adapting to Patient Learning Styles

Imagine that you are a clinical medical assistant in an obstetrics practice. Part of your job is to teach patients, under the supervision of the physician, about what to expect during labor and delivery. Your current task is to assess the knowledge levels and learning styles of three patients. Once you've made your assessment, you will present the physician with a proposal for a plan to teach each patient. For each patient described, determine the patient's dominant learning style and explain how you would suggest teaching each patient so she can best understand.

1. Cora is an active 23-year-old who loves playing tennis and racquetball. She brought her iPod into the exam room, and when you arrive, she is tapping her fingers to the beat she hears through her headphones. You speak with her for a few minutes to determine how much she already understands and what you need to teach her, but she seems a bit restless after only a few minutes.

   Learning style: _____

   Teaching ideas: _____

   _____

   _____

2. Becky is a quiet 25-year-old who, when you tell her that you are going to explain the labor and delivery process, immediately pulls out a notepad, a red pen, and a blue pen. She explains that she wants to take notes so she doesn't forget anything. However, she appears to be distracted when people begin speaking in loud voices in the hall outside the exam room.

   Learning style: _____

   Teaching ideas: _____

   _____

   _____

3. Samantha is a 28-year-old business executive who enjoys talking with other people. She remembers your name from her last visit, and when you enter the room, she greets you by name. She says she has followed the physician's instructions to treat her gestational diabetes and they have helped a lot. In fact, she became interested in this form of diabetes and recently gave a talk about it to a women's group.

   Learning style: _____

   Teaching ideas: _____

   _____

   _____

Understanding Study Skills

Match each of the following definitions with the correct term related to study skills. You will not use all of the terms.

_____ 1. the ability to remember information

_____ 2. the process of breaking down words into recognizable parts

_____ 3. a judgment held by a person or group about members of another group

_____ 4. a process of analyzing and evaluating information to draw a conclusion

_____ 5. the process of planning and controlling the amount of time spent on specific activities to increase efficiency and productivity

_____ 6. a learning technique such as a rhyme, catchphrase, or acronym used to help remember information

_____ 7. a learning disorder characterized by problems processing words

_____ 8. reading with extreme concentration and focus

_____ 9. a person who learns through experiencing and doing activities, such as labs and field trips

_____ 10. the different ways in which people learn

_____ 11. a process by which one initiates, guides, and maintains goal-oriented behavior

_____ 12. a resource that identifies synonyms

_____ 13. a person who learns through seeing visual representations of ideas and concepts, such as charts and videos

_____ 14. a set of words known and used by a person

_____ 15. a conclusion that something is true about a person or group that is made without examining the facts

A. active reading
B. auditory learner
C. critical thinking
D. decoding
E. dyslexia
F. generalization
G. goal
H. kinesthetic learner
I. learning styles
J. mnemonic device
K. motivation
L. retention
M. stereotype
N. thesaurus
O. time management
P. visual learner
Q. vocabulary

Time Management

Time management is an important skill not only for studying, but also for prioritizing tasks at work. Read the scenario below, and then answer the questions that follow to help Tim prioritize his school and work tasks.

Tim is going to school in the evenings to become a registered nurse. To help make ends meet until he can get a job as an RN, he is also working part-time, from 8:00 a.m. to 12:00 p.m., as an administrative assistant at a local clinic. His supervisor has told him that he is welcome to study during slow times at the clinic, as long as it does not interfere with his work.

As Tim drives to the clinic, he is hoping that today will be a slow day. He has a test tonight in his anatomy and physiology class, and he has not had time to study as much as he wants to. He also has a report on diseases of the nervous system due in three days, and he has not even started to research the topic. Tim has promised to meet a friend this afternoon before the A&P class to go over study notes together. However, he isn't sure how useful that will be, since they are meeting in the school's noisy cafeteria.

When Tim arrives at the clinic at 7:55, the phones are already ringing, and he sees several pages in the fax machine. One of the physicians comes in, demanding to know whether Tim has seen a missing patient chart. Several patients have already arrived and are standing around the reception desk, waiting to check in. Another physician walks in with a thick patient chart that he wants Tim to copy and send to a colleague in New York.

1. List the tasks that Tim needs to prioritize and manage.

_____

_____

_____

_____

2. How would you suggest that Tim manage these tasks?

_____

_____

_____

_____

3. What suggestions might you give Tim to help him manage future work and school deadlines?

_____

_____

_____

_____

_____

Fun with Mnemonic Devices

Mnemonic devices are often used by healthcare workers to help them remember important ideas or processes. For example, one common mnemonic device for taking a patient history is the acronym SAMPLE:

Signs and symptoms
Allergies
Medications
Past medical history of injuries or illnesses
Last time the person ate or drank anything
Events that led to the present injury or illness

Other mnemonic devices include rhymes, silly sayings, or even catchphrases, as described in your textbook. You can create a mnemonic device to help you remember just about anything, but the best mnemonic devices are those to which you can relate.

To help improve your study habits, create an expression acronym mnemonic device for the nine note-taking suggestions described in chapter 17. Record your mnemonic device here.

Now create a rhyming mnemonic device to help you remember the steps required to reduce eyestrain, as described in chapter 17. Record your mnemonic device here.

_____

_____

_____

Finally, create a catchphrase mnemonic device to help you remember how to spell the word **mnemonic** *or another word you find difficult to spell. Record your mnemonic device here.*

_____

_____

_____

Critical Thinking in Research

The ability to conduct valid research is useful not just for schoolwork, but also for making good decisions in your everyday life. In some ways, conducting research is much easier today than it was 50 years ago. The Internet has brought thousands of resources literally to our fingertips via computers, tablets, and even smartphones. However, not all Internet sources are the same. The goal of many websites is simply to sell an idea or product. Sites with this goal tend to present only information that will make their point and fail to provide valid facts to back up their claims. Other websites present information that is not well researched. This information may be questionable or even completely wrong. Therefore, it pays to know how to determine whether an Internet source is reliable.

Indications that a website is reliable and credible include the following:

- *The website is sponsored by tax revenue or donations, rather than sales of the product being discussed. Examples: websites for the American Heart Association and the Centers for Disease Control and Prevention*

- *Contact information (street address or e-mail) for the organization associated with the site is available (usually via a "Contact Us" link). Example: the American Cancer Society website*

- *The content on the website is provided or monitored by a professional organization or the federal government. Example: the National Institutes of Health website*

- *The information includes posting dates so that you can tell how recent (or outdated!) the information is. Example: the US Department of Labor's Occupational Safety & Health Administration website*

Use the Internet to research strategies for improving your vocabulary or reading skills, which will supplement information presented in your textbook. List at least three ideas that were not mentioned in the textbook. Provide the source (or sources) where you found each idea and explain how you determined that the websites were reliable and credible.

Ideas: _____

_____

_____

_____

_____

Sources: _____

_____

_____

_____

Clues that these are reliable sources: _____

_____

_____

_____

_____

Reading Practice

The following text is excerpted from the Centers for Disease Control and Prevention's (CDC) information about the Zika virus. Using the techniques for reading difficult or dense passages described in chapter 17, actively read this excerpt. Then summarize the material in your own words.

Zika virus is a single-stranded RNA virus of the Flaviviridae family, genus Flavivirus. Zika virus is transmitted to humans primarily through the bite of an infected *Aedes* species mosquito (*Ae. aegypti* and *Ae. albopictus)*. The mosquito vectors typically breed in domestic water-holding containers; they are aggressive daytime biters and feed both indoors and outdoors near dwellings. Nonhuman and human primates are likely the main reservoirs of the virus, and anthroponotic (human-to-vector-to-human) transmission occurs during outbreaks.

Perinatal, in utero, and possible sexual and transfusion transmission events have also been reported. Zika virus RNA has been identified in asymptomatic blood donors during an ongoing outbreak.

Many people infected with Zika virus are asymptomatic. Characteristic clinical findings are acute onset of fever with maculopapular rash, arthralgia, or conjunctivitis. Other commonly reported symptoms include myalgia and headache. Clinical illness is usually mild with symptoms lasting for several days to a week. Severe disease requiring hospitalization is uncommon and case fatality is low. However, there have been cases of Guillain-Barré syndrome reported in patients following suspected Zika virus infection. Recently, CDC concluded that Zika virus infection during pregnancy is a cause of microcephaly and other severe fetal brain defects. Due to concerns of microcephaly caused by maternal Zika virus infection, fetuses and infants of women infected with Zika virus during pregnancy should be evaluated for possible congenital infection and neurologic abnormalities.

Summary: _____

_____

_____

_____

_____

_____

_____

_____

_____

_____

_____

_____

Chapter 18

Employability Skills

Name _____ Date _____

Matching Professional Terms

Match each of the following definitions with the correct term. You will not use all of the terms.

_____ 1. a letter that accompanies a résumé to provide additional information about the applicant's skills and experience

_____ 2. the process of developing contacts and relationships with people who are interested in your future employment

_____ 3. the ability to change or adjust your attitude and behavior to meet particular needs

_____ 4. the act of making decisions about the best order in which to perform multiple tasks so the most important tasks are completed first

_____ 5. personal characteristics that enable a person to have pleasant, effective interactions with others

_____ 6. the ability to do your job well

_____ 7. an excited and positive attitude that you can bring to your work

_____ 8. the settlement of differences in which each side makes concessions

_____ 9. a skill that helps you interact calmly with coworkers and patients

_____ 10. performing several jobs at the same time

_____ 11. a deep awareness and concern for the suffering of others coupled with the desire to relieve this suffering

_____ 12. the ability to be on time for work, appointments, and any other commitments

_____ 13. the act of identifying with and understanding another person's feelings or situation

_____ 14. a letter written by you to illustrate your personality, passions, and goals for your career

_____ 15. the ability to avoid giving offense through your words and actions

_____ 16. the quality of being honest and having strong moral principles

_____ 17. a document that summarizes your education, work experiences, and other qualifications for employment

_____ 18. term that describes the levels of authority in an organization from the bottom to the top

A. career portfolio
B. chain of command
C. compassion
D. competence
E. compromise
F. conflict resolution
G. cover letter
H. empathy
I. enthusiasm
J. flexibility
K. integrity
L. letter of introduction
M. multitasking
N. networking
O. patience
P. prioritizing
Q. professionalism
R. punctuality
S. résumé
T. soft skills
U. tact

Assess Your Knowledge

Answer the following questions.

1. What is *professionalism* and how does it contribute to employability when looking for a job in a healthcare environment like a hospital, nursing home, or clinic?

   _____

   _____

   _____

   _____

   _____

   _____

   _____

2. How does courteous behavior contribute to employability?

   _____

   _____

   _____

   _____

   _____

   _____

   _____

3. How does leadership ability relate to being a good employee? What are some qualities of a good leader?

   _____

   _____

   _____

   _____

   _____

   _____

   _____

   _____

   _____

(Continued)

4. Healthcare careers generally require employees to work cooperatively with others in a team. Provide several examples of how teamwork is used in healthcare as well as several benefits of using teamwork.

_____

_____

_____

_____

_____

_____

5. In almost every working environment, including healthcare, leaders are required to understand and use conflict resolution techniques. List five potential methods for resolving conflict in the workplace.

_____

_____

_____

_____

_____

_____

6. In the healthcare industry, a positive attitude can be the key to professional success. Provide several examples of how a positive attitude can help you at work.

_____

_____

_____

_____

_____

_____

7. What should be included in a strong career portfolio?

_____

_____

_____

_____

_____

_____

(Continued)

8. Name five sources, people, or groups that can assist you in finding a job.

_____

_____

_____

_____

_____

9. List five things you can do to prepare for a job interview.

_____

_____

_____

_____

_____

10. Now it's time for you to play the role of the employer who is attempting to hire a new employee. Create a list of questions you would ask a potential employee during an interview.

_____

_____

_____

_____

_____

_____

_____

_____

_____

_____

_____

_____

_____

_____

Practicing the Job Interview

Choose two or three of your classmates to form a group. In three or four rounds, depending on the size of your group, you will each ask a hypothetical employee the questions you created in the final part of the "Assess Your Knowledge" activity. One group member will be the interviewee, who is looking for a job. Another group member will be the supervisor, who is asking his or her interview questions. Other group members will act as people who are already employees at the facility. Roles should rotate with each new round, so that everyone has a chance to be the interviewee and supervisor, and so that each group member has a chance to use his or her questions.

After each interview, group members will provide constructive criticism to the interviewee. Everyone involved in the exercise should participate and be professional. Record the constructive criticism you receive in the space provided below.

Constructive criticism: _____

_____

_____

_____

_____

_____

_____

_____

_____

_____

_____

_____

_____

_____

_____

_____

_____

_____

_____

_____

_____

_____

The Résumé

Answer the following questions.

1. What is the purpose of a résumé?

   _____

   _____

   _____

   _____

2. If you are providing a printed, physical copy of your résumé, what guidelines should you follow?

   _____

   _____

   _____

   _____

3. What should be included in the *education* section of your résumé?

   _____

   _____

   _____

   _____

   _____

4. In the *work experience* section of your résumé, what information should you include for each of your jobs?

   _____

   _____

   _____

   _____

5. According to the guidelines in your textbook, list some achievements that you might include in the *honors and activities* section of your résumé.

   _____

   _____

   _____

   _____

Creating a Cover Letter

Follow the steps listed here to create your own cover letter.

Step 1: Search online for some reputable and reliable sources of job listings.

Step 2: Identify some jobs for which you are currently interested in applying. Record some of the jobs you find here. Then choose one on which to focus.

_____

_____

_____

_____

Step 3: Find out as much information as you can about the requirements and responsibilities of the job on which you're going to focus. Record that information here.

_____

_____

_____

_____

Step 4: Using the example provided in Figure 18.8 on page 549 of your textbook, and the information you have recorded here, write a cover letter on a separate sheet of paper. This handwritten first draft can be modified.

Step 5: Get feedback on this first draft from someone whose opinion you trust. Record their constructive criticism here.

_____

_____

_____

_____

Step 6: Make corrections to the initial draft of your letter, and then type the letter on a computer using the same format as the textbook example. Attempt to use the same font on the cover letter as you used on your résumé.

Step 7: Determine whether you need to fill out an application to accompany your résumé. Sometimes the application is available online, but you may need to visit the potential employer and pick up an application in person. If required, complete the application before you provide the cover letter and résumé. If you provide references, make sure you ask the references first before supplying their information.

Word Search

Search the grid of letters below for the terms listed in the word bank.

compassion	empathy	networking	résumé
competence	enthusiasm	patience	tact
compromise	flexibility	prioritizing	teamwork
conflict	integrity	professionalism	
cover letter	multitasking	punctuality	

```
C E P R O M I B W R E X E D B S U T E N
O C N F H Q U N E S I M O R P M O C A R
M N B O P A T I E N C E E C P T M A E Y
P E R U S I E Y M H G N I K R O W T E N
E T O F L E X I B I L I T Y C N T B U A
K E R C O M P O R T A X U N R E V M Y U
R P Z E I U H T G U B T D U L F O S F E
O M I N B S V E C W K Q B R K E A I B T
W O N Y A E C U J Q N U E S I D O L E G
M C Y T I R G E T N I V U E N S D A B N
A U D C T A O N E C O N F L I C T N A I
E H K I C T A T E C O I M S U B I O R K
T R N Q P E A H O J T B S O N R C I D S
A G N M O A C U N I O H E S U N R S F A
T I U N H Q B S O N A T M V A O C S I T
N G N I Z I T I R O I R P O H P X E B I
C O N F U Z K A I L U N A T E G M F A T
O N R E C O J S L A M U T G A E R O S L
M E U B A L O M E O P O H A N I H R C U
A B P U N C T U A L I T Y T U F J P E M
```